MEDICINE IN ENGLAND
DURING THE
REIGN OF GEORGE III

AMS PRESS
NEW YORK

MEDICINE IN ENGLAND
DURING THE
REIGN OF GEORGE III

THE FITZPATRICK LECTURES DELIVERED AT THE ROYAL COLLEGE OF PHYSICIANS
1917-1918

BY
ARNOLD CHAPLIN, M.D. (CANTAB.)
FELLOW OF THE COLLEGE

LONDON
HENRY KIMPTON
263 HIGH HOLBORN, W. C. 1
1919

Library of Congress Cataloging in Publication Data

Chaplin, Arnold, 1864-1944.
Medicine in England during the reign of George III.

Reprint of the 1919 ed. published by H. Kimpton, London, as the Fitzpatrick lectures delivered at the Royal College of Physicians, 1917-1918.
"A list of periodical publications devoted to medicine during the reign of George III": p.
1. Medicine—England—History. 2. Great Britain—History—George III, 1760-1820. 3. Medicine—15th-18th centuries. I. Title. II. Series: The Fitzpatrick lectures; 1917-1918.
R487.C46 1977 610'.942 75-23695
ISBN 0-404-13244-8

Reprinted from an original copy in the collections of the Library of the College of Physicians of Philadelphia, Pa.

From the edition of 1919, London
First AMS edition published in 1977
Manufactured in the United States of America

AMS PRESS INC.
NEW YORK, N.Y.

MEDICINE IN ENGLAND
DURING THE REIGN OF GEORGE III

CHAPTER I

GENERAL CONDITIONS—MEDICAL EDUCATION

THE sixty years of the reign of George III witnessed vast intellectual changes which closed for ever the long period of feudalism. They saw the practical application of methods of thought which had been taking definite shape for the past hundred years. They heard the death-knell of principles which had enthralled and fettered Europe for centuries, and they saw the foundations laid of those conceptions of civil and intellectual liberty which have since governed the world. It was an age of men of predominant genius who assailed with splendid courage the last strongholds of reaction and opposition to human progress; an age in which the principle was firmly established that free enquiry was the only sure road to the advancement of knowledge, toleration of opinion, and liberty of action.

But although this spirit of free enquiry was abroad in the land, and although its cause was championed by some of the mightiest intellects of that or of any other age, for a considerable time its victory hung in the balance, and, in any case, its full fruition was postponed for a number of years. For, in the course of its advance, the spirit of free enquiry met with a most powerful and determined opposition in the shape of a

B

reactionary spirit which stood sullenly at bay in its last defences, and during the last thirty years of the eighteenth century nearly succeeded in wrecking the whole movement. Every artifice that the wit of man could devise to check the march of progress was used by the reactionaries. They suspended the right of "habeas corpus," they prohibited the right of freedom of speech, and the right of freedom of the press, and, by the maintenance of the hateful Test and Corporation Acts, and other repressive measures against those who professed unorthodox faiths and opinions, they practically destroyed all semblance of civil, intellectual, and religious liberty.

Then again this age is, perhaps, better known to us than any other in the annals of our history, and its close proximity to our own will surely enlist a measure of our interest and sympathy. The opulence of its literature has made us familiar with its customs, its manners, its great men, and its great women. The lives led by the people of that time, their formal old-world courtesy, their robustness of character, even their foibles, all appeal to us, and occupy a share of our affections. Finally, the age of George III is adorned by some of the greatest names this country has ever produced. It is hallowed by the memory of Burke, the first of all political philosophers, of Fox, the foremost champion of civil and religious liberty, of the stately Gibbon, of the endearingly simple Goldsmith, of the quartet of great Scotsmen, Hunter, Hume, Adam Smith, and Robertson, and of the commanding and representative personality of Johnson, better known, and dearer to us, perhaps, than any other.

If the foregoing be admitted as a true interpretation of the spirit of the age of George III; if it be granted that this age witnessed great general changes in thought and action, great advances in human progress, and the birth of that social and intellectual state under which we at present live; then it will surely follow that the same processes were in operation in the particular realm of medicine, and produced most important changes therein. It becomes, therefore, a matter of interest and profit to trace these changes in the medical profession, for from such a study evidences will be found of the inception of many customs, methods, and theories which have become accepted facts at the present time.

In order to accomplish this purpose it is proposed to give a description of the state of medicine at this period. After offering some brief preliminary observations concerning the general intellectual conditions which exerted an influence on medical thought in the eighteenth century, the special conditions under which medicine flourished during the reign of George III will be dealt with at some length. This part of the subject will include an enquiry into the state of the medical profession as it existed at that time. It will treat of the position of the Royal College of Physicians; of the facilities for the acquirement of medical knowledge in London and at the Universities; of the rise and progress of the hospitals, the dispensaries, the societies, and the medical press. An account will be given of the work of physicians who contributed to the advance of the knowledge of medicine, pathology, obstetrics, lunacy, and dermatology; of the work of those physicians who advanced general science; and of the personal and mental attributes of those who adorned the medical profession by reason of attainments other than scientific and medical. Space will also be devoted to the development of the medical services of the Navy and Army, for during the age of George III many of the fundamental principles which govern those services at the present day were formulated and instituted. Lastly, some account will be given of the illnesses of some distinguished Georgians, with special reference to the diagnoses made and the treatment administered.

The proper appreciation of the particular quality of medical thought during the age of George III involves a consideration of all thought and literature at that time. The last half of the eighteenth century was an age of transition, in which the human intelligence refused to be satisfied with mere speculations, in which it objected to accept ideas as true on the " ipse dixit " of so-called authority, and in which it evinced an overmastering craving for proof. In the latter half of this century doctrines which had withstood the assaults of ages were seen to crumble and wither when subjected to the unrelenting process of investigation founded on a secure scientific basis. The same scientific method carried the thoughts of men to heights hitherto unscaled, and opened up vistas of knowledge never before conceived. The honour of having wrought this change in thought belongs to the French school, of which the chief exponents were Voltaire, Montesquieu, and Rousseau. These men nurtured and brought to fruition the spirit of free enquiry and toleration, and, although they borrowed the idea from Locke, Hobbes, and others in this country, they are nevertheless entitled to praise for having clothed it with their genius and imagination. The first evidence of a change came in the domain of historical writing. Owing to the influence and incessant labours of Voltaire history for the first time came to be written from a rational standpoint. In his " Le Siècle de Louis XIV " for the first time it was no longer a narration of the trivial acts and peculiarities of kings and captains, but an exhaustive enquiry into the manners, customs, and economic conditions governing the destinies of peoples. After this, almost every branch of literature and thought was involved in the same change, until, in the closing years of the eighteenth century was witnessed the final emancipation of the human intellect, the last struggles of feudalistic principles, and the dawn of civil, intellectual, and religious freedom. This beneficent stream of unfettered thought was, at first, without channels, and with the flood-gates wide open, it bid fair to swamp the very things it was intended to conserve and foster. But as time went on it became more and more directed until, early in the nineteenth century, it was so controlled that its full benefits became manifest in every department of life and thought. In a word, the spirit of free enquiry became universal, and the days of mere speculation were numbered.

When the evolution of medical thought during this epoch is considered, little difficulty is experienced in instituting a parallel with the change that had taken place in intellectual Europe. Until the end of the eighteenth century the spirit of scientific enquiry and the desire to appeal to facts ascertained by experiment did not influence medical thought to any great extent. Harvey, the glory of the College of Physicians, was so in advance of his times that he was doomed to wait a century for that suitable soil on which his seed could come to fruition. Indeed, the conclusion is warranted that medical thought during the first half of the eighteenth century accomplished scarcely anything that has withstood the test of time. The theories of medical science promulgated at this time were often the results of metaphysical speculations, and little or no attempt was made to submit them to the supreme test of scientific proof. For this reason the "Systems," raised up with so much labour, and at the expense of such great philosophical ability, were soon swept away when tested by the experimental method.

It is not proposed to deal at any considerable length with the various Systems which arose during the first half of the eighteenth century, and, for a time, exerted a certain influence over medical thought. Although they may be interesting as landmarks and signposts on the road of physiological and chemical progress, yet, since they were founded, for the most part, on mere speculation, they often retarded a just conception of the principles of medicine. Some of these Systems were entirely new, while others were of a composite variety, and made up of the most likely elements of former Systems. The "Animism" of Stahl, the "Æther" of Hoffmann, the "Solidism" of Cullen, the "Iatro-Chemical," the "Iatro-Physical," and the "Old Vienna" schools, all had their votaries and enjoyed a brief popularity. But the illuminating teaching of Harvey and Sydenham had fallen upon deaf ears, and the doctors were still engaged in speculating in the quiet of their studies, instead of seeking for information in the book of nature.[1]

After giving due attention to these various Systems it must be confessed that one rises from the task with a feeling of sadness—sadness that such powerful intellects wasted their abilities on work calculated so little to contribute to the real advancement of medical knowledge. Indeed, to express shortly our view of the effects produced upon medicine by the Systems, a passage from Lord Morley's "Voltaire" might be adopted with but slight substitution of words. "For all the Systems we see only dismal tracts of medical darkness, we hear only the humming of the doctors as they serve forth, to men thirsting after knowledge, the draff of a medical superstition."

The comparative absence of medical advancement during the first half of the eighteenth century can scarcely cause astonishment if the particular education and environment of physicians at that time be taken into account. Those who championed the new scientific method of enquiry were never weary of pointing out

[1] It is not, of course, intended to convey the impression that the work of some of the authors of the "Systems" was valueless from the point of view of physiology and chemistry, for Stahl, von Helmont, and Sylvius were pioneers in these subjects. It is medicine only that is referred to in the above passage.

that much of the inability of thinkers to advance, and many of the misconceptions that had arisen concerning the fundamental principles of life were largely due to the particular teaching then in vogue. They pointed out that a system of teaching which directed mental activities to the fixed and the past was not conducive to an intellectual training for the purpose of advancing on new and, therefore, untrodden paths of thought. If this be true, there can be no doubt that physicians, during the early years of the reign of George III, lacked, as a rule, that particular kind of training, for they were largely under the influence of this special form of teaching. In many of them erudition in classical attainments far outweighed their eminence in medicine and formed, indeed, their chief claim to distinction. Their special mental training encouraged them to place more reliance upon speculative theorising concerning disease than upon the meaning of facts and conditions observed at the bedside and on the post-mortem table.

But a change for the better was close at hand. Early in the reign of George III the work of Morgagni began to produce an effect upon medical thought in England, and soon many physicians were engaged in obtaining a real knowledge of disease from the study of morbid conditions found after death. The logical consequence of the work of Morgagni found expression in the labours of Baillie and Bîchat, both of whom carried the subject forward. These prominent men were the real fathers of modern pathology and medicine. They occupied positions similar to those of Voltaire and Montesquieu in thought, Burke in politics, and Newton in natural philosophy. They were bold innovators who swept away an ancient order of things which had long cumbered the ground, and defied advance. They established, on lines never since departed from, the only rational study of disease. Our debt to them can scarcely be expressed in words.

THE CONDITION OF THE MEDICAL PROFESSION

Having thus summarised the general state of medical thought as it existed at the beginning of the reign of George III, it now becomes necessary to study the more intimate conditions found in the medical profession at that time.

During the reign the medical profession was divided into three grades: physicians, surgeons, and apothecaries. In London, and for seven miles around, these three divisions were governed respectively by the College of Physicians, the Corporation of Surgeons, and the Society of Apothecaries. But beyond this area none of these bodies exercised any very effective control over its members and its privileges. It came to pass, therefore, that many practitioners resided in the provinces who owed no allegiance to those bodies, and often possessed no legal title to practise either medicine or surgery.

It is difficult to arrive at any correct estimate of the actual numbers of practitioners in England at this time, for although the registers of the three licensing bodies can be consulted, they contain a small proportion only of the total. There is, however, one important source of information from which a fairly accurate estimate of the numbers engaged in practice can be obtained. In 1779 Dr. Samuel Foart Simmons, physician to St. Luke's Hospital, published a Medical Register.[1] This was the first attempt to gather into one volume particulars of the medical profession and its activities. Unfortunately only three issues were made, but in the last, which appeared in 1783, data are found from which an estimate of the numerical strength of practitioners resident in England can be calculated. From an investigation of this invaluable book, only a few copies of which are known to exist in London, it is found that in 1782,

[1] "The Medical Register," 1779-80-83.

4459 medical men were resident in England and Wales, to serve a population estimated at 7,814,827 souls, or one medical man for every 1752 people. Of this number, 774 doctors were resident in London, with an estimated population of 650,845, or one medical man to every 840 inhabitants. The subject of overcrowding in the medical profession has been ventilated frequently of late years, but when the ratios just given are compared with those obtaining at the present day no very marked difference will be found. At the present time about 25,000 practitioners in England and Wales serve a population of about 36,000,000, or one to every 1440 people, while in London about 6500 doctors attend about 4,500,000 people, or one to every 705 inhabitants. The author of "A Picture of the College of Physicians"[1] estimated that in 1817 London, with a population of 1,100,000, had in residence 1098 doctors, or one to every 1000 people. Nor can it be said that the scale of remuneration for medical services has altered to any considerable extent. Physicians in those days charged a guinea, at a time when the purchasing power of the sovereign was far greater than it is now. Indeed, it may be stated with safety that a relatively larger number of physicians secured a handsome competence from the practice of medicine in the reign of George III than is the case at the present day, while some, such as Lettsom, Warren, Simmons, and Battie realised large fortunes.

According to the "Medical Register" for 1783 London contained 149 physicians, 274 surgeons, and 351 apothecaries. This return, however, takes no account of many who, owing to the laxness of supervision, sold drugs and practised surreptitiously without any proper authorisation, and the same remark applies with greater force to the provinces. The College, jointly with the Master and Wardens of the Society of Apothecaries, had the power of supervision over drugs sold by

1 "A Picture of the Royal College of Physicians," 1817.

apothecaries, but towards the latter part of the eighteenth century a new order had arisen which, as will be seen, made it necessary to recast the laws and regulations governing the apothecaries. This new order was the druggists, and over these neither the College of Physicians nor the Society of Apothecaries possessed any jurisdiction.

An investigation of the composition of the College of Physicians, and of the parts of London favoured by those belonging to it during this reign, is of considerable interest. In 1746 the College was composed of 54 Fellows and 24 Licentiates. Of these 47 resided in the City and 14 in the West End.[1] In 1782 there were 43 Fellows and 74 Licentiates, of whom 35 lived in the City and 42 in the West.[2] The migration from the City to the West had now begun to be marked, and in 1817, out of 89 Fellows and 224 Licentiates, 32 only lived in the City, while 105 practised in the West.[3] From this time the exodus from the City progressed steadily, until at the present day two Fellows only remain to uphold the honour of the College in the heart of the greatest city in the world.

An examination of the number of Fellows and Licentiates admitted is also instructive. From 1760 to 1820 inclusive, 128 Fellows were created, or an average of 2.1 per annum, and during the same period 416 Licentiates were admitted, or an average of 6.9 per annum. During the last thirty years of the reign the influx of Licentiates became pronounced, and at the end of the reign they outnumbered the Fellows in a proportion of nearly three to one.[4] This influx of Licentiates must be

[1] See "An Address to the College," 1747.

[2] See "The Medical Register," 1783.

[3] "A Picture of the College," 1817.

[4] The above calculation has been made from Munk's "Roll of the College of Physicians." It should be remembered that the Licentiates in the days of George III did not correspond to those holding the same diploma at the present day, but rather to the Members of the College of our times.

attributed to the rising influence of the Edinburgh school, which was nearing its zenith. A large number of men were taught in Edinburgh, and those who came to seek their fortune in England were obliged, by the laws in force regarding physicians, to become Licentiates of the College.

MEDICAL LAWS AND REGULATIONS

Attention must now be paid to a consideration of the laws and regulations under which the medical profession worked at this period. No central authority possessing powers under Parliamentary Acts existed, but the three corporate bodies of the College of Physicians, the Corporation of Surgeons, and the Society of Apothecaries respectively exercised jurisdiction over physicians, the surgeons, and the apothecaries. But even then the power to assert authority by these bodies was limited and often exhibited in a lax manner. As might be supposed, their charters, granted in a bygone age, were ill-adapted to new and constantly changing conditions. They referred rather to the profession resident in London, and contained no strict provisions for the control of those of their members who resided in the provinces. The College of Physicians possessed ample authority over all physicians engaged in practice in London, and no physician could pursue his vocation in the metropolis and seven miles around without a licence from the College, after having been duly examined. Further, by the first Statute (14 & 15 Henry VIII, c. 5) which confirmed the original Charter, the College was given power to examine and grant licences to all physicians in England, with the important exceptions of graduates in medicine of Oxford and Cambridge. Over them it had no jurisdiction so long as they practised in the provinces. Previous to the granting of the first Charter of the College, the right had been conceded to the Bishop of London and the Dean of St. Paul's, with the assistance of physicians and surgeons, to examine and grant licences to those wishing to engage in practice. The same right was also given to a Bishop or his Vicar-General in the provinces. Even so late as 1687 some Bishops continued to exercise this right, and the practice was not given up until the College had issued a warning on the subject to each Bishop. In addition to its other powers, the College was possessed of the right of entering apothecaries' shops in order to inspect the drugs offered for sale.

In much the same way the Corporation of Surgeons and the Society of Apothecaries exercised jurisdiction over members of their bodies, but the control was far less efficient than that of the College. In London it might be described as fairly effective, but in the provinces it left much to be desired. This failure of control, especially so far as it regarded the Society of Apothecaries, was due to the fact that it had no authority over those who were not members of the Society. Consequently a large body of practitioners came into existence, and soon caused considerable alarm. These men were not members of any legally constituted body, they held no diploma entitling them to practise medicine and surgery, but, notwithstanding, they carried on their business without let or hindrance. Soon they formed the majority of the medical profession, but no power existed by which they could be brought under proper control. In London these buccaneers of the profession could be dealt with in an effective manner, but not so in the provinces. According to John Mason Good, these men were merely druggists who, in addition to selling drugs, compounded and dispensed medicines and practised medicine and surgery. They sold pure drugs to the apothecary, but reserved the impure drugs for their own use. They were unversed in Latin, and could not, therefore, read prescriptions.[1] They first made their appearance towards the end of the seventeenth century, and, by the end of the eighteenth century, they had become so numerous that it was felt on all sides that something should be attempted to bring them under some sort of control.

The result of this incursion of unqualified and ignorant men into the medical profession was the passing of the Apothecaries Act in 1815, but before this could be accomplished public opinion had to be roused concerning the danger. In this agitation for a better state of things the names of John Mason Good and George Man Burrows stand out prominently, and it was owing entirely to their powerful advocacy that the reform was brought about. The former founded the "Pharmaceutic Association" in 1794, while the latter was responsible for the "Association of Surgeon Apothecaries," both societies being devoted to the improvement of the position of that branch of the profession. If they received no encouragement, at least they met with no active opposition, from the Colleges of Physicians and Surgeons, and soon the labours of the two Associations bore fruit. On August 1st, 1815, the "Apothecaries Act" became law, and for the first time in the history of medicine in this country, cognisance was taken of the principle that all those who practised must first be properly qualified.

By the provisions of the "Apothecaries Act," all those who kept an apothecary's shop were required to pass an examination before examiners appointed by the Society of Apothecaries, and all candidates for the examination were required to give proof of having served five years as apprentices. The Master and Wardens of the Society were empowered to enter any apothecary's shop in England and Wales and to impose fines if impure drugs

[1] For a full account of this movement see "History of Medicine so far as it relates to the Apothecary," John Mason Good, 1796, and various tracts by G. M. Burrows.

were found. Finally, no apothecary could recover debts in a court of law unless he possessed a licence to practise.[1]

There can be no doubt that the passing of this Act marked an immense advance in the regulations for the control of the profession, and it was the forerunner of all subsequent Acts. It had, however, its defects, and it would have been well had the two Colleges enquired more closely regarding the consequences of this Act. What was its effect? At a stroke the education of about three-fourths of those who contemplated entering the medical profession was placed under the entire control of the Society of Apothecaries through legal powers granted by Parliament. The Colleges had no voice in the matter of determining the scope of medical education, and could deal only with those belonging to their own bodies. It must be admitted that their policy was somewhat short-sighted, for it would have been a comparatively easy matter to adjust their relations with the Society of Apothecaries in such a manner that a share of the control conferred by Parliament would have fallen to their lot. As it was, the Colleges were shut out from all participation in the control of the education of the greater number of the profession, and many years had to elapse before they regained their power.

MEDICAL EDUCATION

Consideration may now be given to the facilities existing for the acquirement of medical knowledge during this period, and to the standard deemed necessary. At this time the three capitals of the British Isles were the only centres at which medical education could be obtained, and, so far as regards the number of students, London and Edinburgh were far in advance of Dublin. In London seven general hospitals were established where a knowledge of medicine could be obtained. At

[1] For the detailed provisions of the "Apothecaries Act" see "The Statutes," 55 George III C. 194, and "Parliamentary History," 1815.

Guy's, St. Thomas's, and the London hospitals, systematic courses of lectures in the Theory of Medicine, Materia Medica, Chemistry, and Clinical Medicine were given, but in most of the other hospitals the teaching was sadly neglected. Too often the members of the medical and surgical staffs considered it to be no part of their duty to give instruction except to a few favoured pupils from whom they exacted a premium for the privilege.

As a rule, the subjects of Medicine, Materia Medica, Anatomy, and Chemistry were taught at schools and lectures supported by private enterprise, of which there were many in the metropolis at this time. In the "Medical Register" for 1783[1] a page is devoted to a list of lectures, and of the nineteen given there all were supported by private enterprise with the exceptions of those at the London, St. Thomas's, and Guy's Hospitals. Indeed, it appears that Dr. George Fordyce of St. Thomas's, Dr. William Saunders of Guy's, and Dr. James Maddox of the London, were the only physicians who gave systematic courses of lectures at the institutions to which they were attached. In the same manner the subject of midwifery was taught by means of private lectures given by Denman, Osborne, Orme, John Clarke, and David Davis. Prominent among these private lecturers was Dr. George Fordyce, who lectured for thirty years on Physic, Materia Medica, and Chemistry at his house in Essex Street, Strand. He was assiduous and unremitting in his work; beginning at seven in the morning, he delivered three lectures, each lasting an hour, on six days in the week, and probably nearly all the students coming to London at this period passed through his hands.[2] The teaching of Anatomy was

[1] See the "Medical Register" 1783, and the Appendix to this volume.

[2] For an excellent memoir of Dr. George Fordyce see the "Gentleman's Magazine," June, 1802, from the pen of his friend and colleague Dr. W. C. Wells.

carried on chiefly at the school in Windmill Street, where the brilliant abilities of the two Hunters, Hewson, Cruikshank, Baillie, and Wilson made it deservedly famous. Mr. John Shelden, Dr. R. Maclaurin, and Mr. Blizzard also taught Anatomy at their respective houses with considerable success.

After a student had attended lectures and the practice of a hospital for a sufficient length of time, which varied at different periods, he was free to present himself for examination at the Corporation of Surgeons, or the Society of Apothecaries, and if he satisfied the examiners he was granted a diploma. Often, however, he did not follow this course, but after studying medicine and surgery betook himself to the provinces and began practice without any diploma. He was quite secure, and no law could reach him so long as he remained away from London.

When, however, a student decided to practise as a physician the course to be pursued was different and far more exacting. It was necessary for him to obtain a degree in some University, and, in due time, to submit himself to the examination for Licentiates at the College of Physicians. This course was obligatory for all physicians, with the exception of those engaged in practice in the provinces who were in possession of the M.D. degree of either Oxford or Cambridge. The holders of these degrees were exempted by statute from being obliged to become Licentiates so long as they practised in the provinces. But the College of Physicians exercised no very strict supervision over physicians beyond the London area, and many were actively engaged in practice who were not in possession of the M.D. degree of either Oxford or Cambridge. From all accounts, the examination for the Licence of the College, which was conducted in Latin, was thorough and searching. It not only established the fact that a successful candidate was learned in the principles of medicine, but it proved also that he was a man of considerable erudition and culture. The examination for the Candidates for the Fellowship was precisely the same as that for the Licentiate, and the College could justly claim that the members of their body were men of far higher mental attainments than those of the Corporation of Surgeons, and the Society of Apothecaries.

At the Universities of Oxford and Cambridge the Professors of Physic and Anatomy delivered courses of lectures, and so also did the Professors or Readers of Botany and Chemistry, but the reading of these lectures appears to have been of a somewhat perfunctory nature, and no practical instruction appears to have been given. Those who intended, therefore, to become physicians settled at centres where the serious study of medicine could be prosecuted, and, except for the purpose of fulfilling the requirements of the Universities in the matter of a medical degree, were hardly ever in residence. During the early years of the reign, London, Edinburgh, Dublin, and Aberdeen were the only places in this country where a medical education could be acquired, and none of them enjoyed a reputation sufficient to attract a large number of those who proposed to become physicians. Many, therefore, proceeded to the various schools on the Continent, and it was only in the latter years of the reign that the excellence of the medical teaching in London, and especially in Edinburgh, attracted large numbers of those who desired to perfect themselves in the art of medicine.

At the sister Universities the regulations relating to medical degrees differed, and are, indeed, difficult to follow with any exactness. According to the author of "An address to the College,"[1] the method of procedure in granting medical degrees at Oxford was as follows. No person could be admitted to the honour

[1] See "An Address to the College," 1747, pp. 7–9. This account appears to be the most accurate, and has, therefore, been adopted.

of a doctor's degree in medicine until he had been a member of the University for fourteen years, and had complied with all the exercises required. In other words, he was expected to become a Bachelor of Arts in four years, a Master in seven years, a Bachelor of Medicine in ten years, and a Doctor in fourteen years. The principle, therefore, of a degree in arts before proceeding to one in medicine was established. For the B.A. degree candidates were required to defend questions in logic, grammar, rhetoric, and moral philosophy; to be examined in the same subjects, and all the examinations and exercises were conducted in Latin. For the M.A. degree the candidate was again required to defend questions in the subjects for the B.A., and, in addition, questions in Natural and Moral Philosophy. Lastly, he was required to pass an examination in Geometry, Metaphysics, Optics, Physics, History, Geography, Chronology, Latin, and Greek. At Cambridge the exercises for the same degree appear to have been similar, but perhaps more latitude was allowed to candidates in specialising in particular subjects. Now, whatever may have been the way in which these exercises were kept in the letter, and many asserted that they were a mere farce, there can be no doubt that in the spirit they contained the framework of a comprehensive intellectual training. Indeed, those who relied on the system at the two Universities as the best preliminary course for those intending to become physicians could point with truth to the regulations in force to prove their argument. For the M.B. degree the candidate was expected to defend two subjects in physic for two hours, and to oppose two others for a like period. In 1760, according to Dr. Wells, the Act for the degree of Bachelor of Medicine consisted of reading the Aphorisms of Hippocrates.[1] However that may be, the candidate was obliged to go through a

[1] See "A Letter to Lord Kenyon," p. 109 note. Wells.

course of anatomy before proceeding to keep the Act. For the M.D. degree the candidate was required to explain a whole book of Galen in six extempore or three written lectures.

At Cambridge perhaps a somewhat more pronounced attempt was made to impart medical knowledge by means of lectures, and some of the professors appear to have performed their functions with some little show of energy. The degree of Bachelor of Medicine could be taken six years after admission, provided that the candidate had kept nine terms at the University. Two public disputes had to be maintained in Latin by the candidate. One question was chosen by the candidate and the other by the professor. The candidate then read a thesis on his own question, and defended it and the professor's question against the arguments of the professor and other doctors present. Finally, the professor read his "Determination" in Latin. This proceeding was conducted in the public schools, and, as a rule, many spectators were present.[1] The degree of M.D. could be taken five years after the M.B. degree, and the exercises required were on the same lines as those for the M.B. Dr. Wells states that originally the candidate was obliged to oppose another candidate, but that this regulation was abrogated on the payment of a fine of twenty shillings. He also asserted that the professor's question could be obtained by the candidate at any time, however long, before the Act was kept.[2] At Cambridge and Oxford a doctor's degree in medicine was sometimes given by "Royal Mandate," and apparently it was not always obligatory to proceed in Arts before taking the M.B. degree, although this course was generally pursued. Besides the degrees of M.B. and M.D. the Universities granted a "Licence to Practise." Professor Haviland, however, in his evi-

[1] See "The Medical Register," 1780.

[2] See "A Letter to Lord Kenyon," p. 109 note. Wells.

dence before the Select Committee of the House of Commons in 1834, stated that few took the "Licence to Practise." He also stated that the examination was more practical than that for the M.B., and that, since the possession of the M.B. degree sometimes disqualified from holding a Fellowship, the "Licence to Practise" was taken in preference.[1] The foregoing then is a picture of the course of education followed by many of those who desired to become physicians. The tendency of that education was in the direction of general culture, and accounts for the high order of intellectual capacity which was such a prominent feature of the College of Physicians in those days.

In other Universities the same spirit prevailed, but in many of them the insistence on the acquirement of general knowledge was far less pronounced, and more facilities were afforded for becoming versed in the principles and practice of medicine. Especially was this the case at Edinburgh and Leyden, whither many physicians during the reign repaired for the purpose of undertaking the serious study of medicine.

HOSPITALS AND DISPENSARIES

In close association with the facilities for the acquirement of medical knowledge was the rise and development of the hospitals and dispensaries in London and the provinces; truly one of the most remarkable features in the medical history of the reign. When George III ascended the throne in 1760, London possessed seven general hospitals, two asylums, and six special hospitals, but not a single dispensary. So far back as 1696 an attempt had been made by the College of Physicians to establish a dispensary for the benefit of those who were too poor to purchase pure drugs,

[1] See Haviland's evidence before the Select Committee of the House of Commons, appointed to enquire concerning Medical Education. "Parliamentary Papers," 1834, pp. 243–263.

but after a time the project fell into abeyance.[1] With that exception no dispensary existed in the metropolis until 1770, when the General Dispensary in Aldersgate Street was founded. This was followed by the Westminster Dispensary in 1774, and between that date and the close of the reign in 1820 no less than thirty-four dispensaries and three hospitals came into being, of which eighteen remain in active work at the present day.

In the provinces the same conditions prevailed. Before 1760 sixteen hospitals and one asylum represented all the public institutions in existence for the treatment of the sick poor. But during the reign no less than forty-five hospitals, thirty-six dispensaries, and eight asylums were founded in various parts of England, with the result that accommodation for the treatment of disease amongst the poor became ample.[2]

The need for increased facilities for the medical treatment of the poor of growing England, and the wider conceptions in vogue concerning the duties of the rich towards the poor, no doubt were largely responsible for the foundation of the hospitals and dispensaries. Many of these institutions, however, owed their origin to the insistent demands of energetic physicians, who, supported by their influential friends, desired a field for clinical work. At that time, physicians of great ability were beginning to flock to England, especially from the rising school of Edinburgh. The possibilities of obtaining positions where they could found professional reputations as teachers were few, and the staffs of existing hospitals were limited and

[1] In this connection mention should be made of Garth's poem "The Dispensary," in which the characters and peculiarities of many of the Fellows of the College of that day are painted with much wit and humour.

[2] For further information concerning dispensaries see "Laws and Plans of Dispensaries," 1765-1811, and "History Design, and Present State of Public Charities." A. Highmore, 1810.

exclusive. In this difficulty the more enterprising spirits threw themselves with ardour into the project, and so it came to pass that the new hospitals and dispensaries were staffed by some of the ablest and most enlightened physicians in the country. The names of Fothergill, Lettsom, James Sims, Hulme, Johnston, Simmons, Wells, and Willan are prominently connected with this movement, and some of the dispensaries in London, such as the " General," the " Westminster," and the " Public," soon became centres for teaching, and the excellence of the clinical instruction attracted many students. A particular interest attaches to the " Public Dispensary " in Carey Street, for it was there that Robert Willan and his pupil Thomas Bateman prosecuted their researches in Dermatology, and gave to the world the first attempt to classify skin diseases from an anatomical standpoint.

Further evidence of medical activity in this reign is found in the rise of the numerous societies devoted to the advancement of medicine. Probably the earliest society of this kind of which we have any record was one founded by Glisson about 1650, and mentioned in his work on Rickets. The next was the Society of Naval Surgeons, which began its career in 1746. This society engaged Mr. Sharp to deliver lectures on surgical operations, and met at a house in Covent Garden. Sharp was soon succeeded by William Hunter, who continued the course for several years. In 1752 a Medical Society of Physicians was founded, chiefly owing to the energy of Fothergill, and met at the Mitre Tavern. The next to be formed was the " Society of Licentiate Physicians " in 1764 by Fothergill and Alexander Russell. Licentiates of the College only were eligible for election, and the meetings were held at "Old Slaughter's Coffee House," but once a quarter the members dined at the "Crown and Anchor." In 1767, at the instigation of Dr. Heberden, the " Meetings of the

College of Physicians" were begun, and between that date and 1820 six volumes of transactions were issued. 1771 saw the foundation of the "Guy's Physical Society" by Dr. William Saunders, and the same year witnessed the establishment of the Physico-Medical Society. The Medical Society was founded in 1773, and in the following year the "Middlesex Hospital Society" began its career. Mr. John Shelden formed a Medical Society in 1779, which met at his house in Great Queen Street, and in 1762, owing to the efforts of Dr. Simmons, Dr. Fordyce, and John Hunter, the Society for the Improvement of Medical Knowledge was established, the meetings being held at "Old Slaughter's Coffee House." Fordyce was also responsible for the foundation of the "Lyceum Medicis Londinense" in 1785. Finally, the "Medical and Philosophical Society of St. Bartholomew's," renamed in 1832 the "Abernethian,"[1] was formed in 1795, the "Medico-Chirurgical" in 1805, and the "Hunterian" in 1819. A Society of Physicians to Dispensaries met in the Borough about 1780, but the exact date of its foundation is uncertain.[2]

It will thus be seen that twelve medical societies were formed during the reign of George III, and three only before that period. Many of them came to an end after a few years of usefulness, but six remain and are flourishing at the present time. Among those who did so much to encourage the formation of these London medical societies the names of Fothergill, Simmons, Lettsom, Fordyce, and William Hunter must be for ever honoured. They toiled, not unsuccessfully, for the advancement of medicine, and for a wider medical polity where men holding diverse opinions could meet and exchange their views.

[1] For an account of the "Abernethian" Society, see St. Bart's Hosp. Reports, Vol. IV, by Dr. Rowland Combs.

[2] This statement rests on the authority of Leonard Gillespie, whose diary will be found in the "Admiralty Medical Journals," Admiralty Series, Public Record Office.

In the provinces also three medical societies were formed during the reign. The first one being the Colchester Medical Society in 1774. This was followed by the Plymouth Medical Society in 1794, and the Leicester Medical Society in 1800, but previous to the formation of these three societies there is no record to be found of any similar society existing in the provinces. To complete the review of the establishment of medical societies, it remains to be said that towards the end of the eighteenth century six medical benevolent societies were founded in the provinces and one in London, all of which are flourishing at the present day.[1]

THE ROYAL COLLEGE OF PHYSICIANS

The position of the College of Physicians with regard to medical progress must now claim attention. This enquiry embraces the history of the great contest between the Fellows and the Licentiates; it also involves an investigation of the powers conferred by Charter upon the College and the spirit in which they were applied.

The great contest in the College between the Fellows and the Licentiates definitely began in 1752, although the first mutterings of the coming storm were heard as far back as 1746. From that date it dragged on its weary length for more than eighty years, sometimes waxing and sometimes waning, but never really ceasing. Small advances occupied decades for their attainment, and it was not until the beginning of the reign of Queen Victoria that the College could see its way to concede the main great principle for which the Licentiates had contended. For a long time the College was apparently

[1] Much of the information concerning the history of the medical societies will be found in the "Medical Register," 1789–93. See also "Hunterian Oration" by Dr. Newton Pitt, "Lancet," 1896, Vol. I, and Mr. D'Arcy Power's Account. I have also to acknowledge my indebtedness to Dr. Clippingdale, who has allowed me to read his invaluable MSS. dealing with that subject.

content to accept the existing order of things, and appeared little disposed to move in the direction of any change. Some of the Licentiates, however, were active in their efforts for what they held to be a salutary reform. Amongst these reformers may be mentioned the names of Fothergill, Archer, Wells, Ferris, and Stanger, and no small part of the advancement made in medico-political spheres was due to the persistent advocacy of these men. In season and, it must also be admitted, often out of season, they urged upon the College the necessity for reform. To their unwearied perseverance we owe it that the College now rests on the sure foundations of justice and liberality towards the three estates over which it exercises jurisdiction.

What was this contest between the Fellows and the Licentiates ? It arose in this way. The Charter of the incorporation of the College, and the Statutes of 14 and 15, Henry VIII, gave the whole control over the practice of physic into the hands of the College with the exception that Doctors of Medicine of Oxford and Cambridge might practice in the provinces free from that control. In 1555 the College saw fit to pass a bye-law limiting the number of its Fellows, and at the same time instituted the grade of Licentiates. In addition to these enactments, the practice had grown up in the College of electing to the Fellowship only those who possessed the degree of Doctor of Medicine from the Universities of Oxford and Cambridge. It is not very clear when the bye-law embodying this principle was put into operation, but is was probably not before 1575. By this practice, therefore, which became the established rule of the College, the whole of its government was placed in the hands of those who were Doctors of Medicine of Oxford and Cambridge, and Doctors of Medicine of other Universities, unless they could become incorporated with Oxford or Cambridge, were relegated to the grade of Licentiates, without any prospect of ever becoming Fellows, or of having any voice in the government of the College. The examination at the College for a Licentiate was precisely the same as that for a Candidate for the Fellowship. Outside the walls of the College the Licentiate enjoyed the same privileges and distinction as a Fellow, but within the College he was beneath them. This was the position which gave rise to the contest between the Fellows and the Licentiates. Holding that they were the equals of the Fellows, in that they had performed the same exercises, they claimed that they should be admitted to the examination for the Candidates for the Fellowship with its rights and privileges.

The contest really began with the demand of Isaac Schomberg to be admitted to the examination for the Candidates for the Fellowship. Schomberg had, in defiance of the Statutes, practised in London as a physician, and was summoned in 1746 by the Censors' Board to present himself for the examination for the Licentiates. This he refused to do, but in 1747, having been entered at Trinity College, Cambridge, he asked to be allowed to practise until he should obtain the M.D. degree. This the College refused, and interdicted him from practice until he had given satisfaction. In 1749 Schomberg obtained the M.D. degree by Royal Mandate, and then applied to be examined, but the College refused this until such time that the interdiction was removed. He then offered an apology which was accepted by some but not by all. In 1750 he demanded to be examined for the Candidate for the Fellowship in virtue of his M.D. degree. He was allowed to sit, and was adjudged competent, but this decision was negatived by a majority, and he was refused admission. Schomberg then took his case to the Law Courts, but met with no success, the Court holding that the College had full power to do as they thought fit. However, in 1765 he was admitted a Licentiate, and in 1771 a Fellow.

He even attained to the dignity of being a Censor in 1773 and 1778.[1] This case called forth Sir William Browne's "Vindication of the College," which he intended to read as a reply to the contentions of Schomberg had the "Visitors" decided to hear the case. It is perhaps fortunate that no such occasion arose for reading this piece, for it is the most vain and pedantic effusion that ever proceeded from the pen of that singular personality.[2]

After this, three acts performed by the College contributed largely to the accentuation of the differences between the Fellows and the Licentiates. They were as follows :—

1. Subsequent to the year 1752 the practice of summoning the Licentiates to the College meetings was abandoned. 2. The College passed in 1752 the "Statutum Alterum de Candidatis," in which it was stated in unmistakable language that no person could become a Fellow unless he held the degree of Doctor of Medicine of either Oxford or Cambridge. 3. In 1765 the Statutes and Bye-Laws of the College, after having been revised, were printed for the use of the College officers, thus rendering them available for the purposes of investigation.

These acts, but particularly the "Statutum Alterum de Candidatis," were the cause of the recrudescence of the controversy in 1765. Two parties were formed. The Licentiates maintained that there were many belonging to their body who, although they possessed no Doctorate degree from the sister Universities, were nevertheless thoroughly fitted by education and medical attainments to adorn the Fellowship of the College. On the other hand, the thick and thin supporters of the existing order were convinced that no man who had not been educated at either Oxford or Cambridge

[1] For the Case of Schomberg, see "Minutes of the Proceedings Relating to Dr. Schomberg," 1754.

[2] 'A Vindication of the College." Sir W. Browne, 1753.

could be worthy of the honour of the Fellowship. The Licentiates held that the action of the College in excluding them was contrary to the spirit of the Statutes in virtue of which the College exercised authority and jurisdiction. They pointed out that anyone holding a degree in medicine from a foreign University could become incorporated at either Oxford or Cambridge on that degree, and could in that way gain admission to the Fellowship. They also urged that the curriculum at Oxford and Cambridge scarcely existed for medical students; that the study of medicine in the sister Universities was a farce which could be performed in four years by anyone holding an M.A. degree, at the expense of attending a few lectures. This, no doubt, was true with regard to the teaching of medicine, but it must be remembered that both Oxford and Cambridge offered considerable facilities for the acquirement of a wide culture. All those intending to study medicine were obliged to graduate in Arts, and the scope of the course instituted for the degrees of Bachelor and Master of Arts has already been described.

To all these contentions of the Licentiates the College turned a deaf ear. They asserted that they knew the form of teaching at Oxford and Cambridge, but were ignorant of the kind of study required at other Universities in the United Kingdom both for Arts and Medicine. They were satisfied that the only way, in fact, to maintain a high standard of culture and medical knowledge at the College was to admit those only to the Fellowship who possessed the passport of an education gained at either Oxford or Cambridge.

The pen was largely used by the opposing sides, and "letters," "addresses," and "reflections" for and against were issued.[1] So high ran the feeling that in

[1] Among these, see "A Letter from a Physician in Town," 1753. "An Attempt to Reconcile All Differences," 1753. "An Address to the College," 1747. "Letters Addressed to the College." Faulkner, 1829.

1767 the Licentiates attempted by force to attend the College meetings, and on one occasion actually succeeded in forcing the doors. The literary value of these pamphlets is not of a high order, but exceptions must be made of the "General View" of Ferris, and the weighty "Letter to Lord Kenyon" by Dr. Wells,[1] both of which are even models of what such polemical writing should be. In another class is "The Battle of the Wigs,"[2] a mock heroic poem in imitation of Garth's "Dispensary," by Bonnell Thornton, wherein the disputes between the two factions are described and ridiculed.

The whole matter was then tested in the Courts in the famous actions of "Rex *v.* Dr. Askew," and "Rex *v.* The College."[3] These trials took place in 1768–9 and 1769–71. They were heard at great length, and arose out of an application by Dr. Letch, Dr. Archer, and Dr. Fothergill for a rule calling upon the Censors to show by what authority they exercised their powers and functions. The cases were heard by Lord Mansfield, Mr. Justice Aston, and Mr. Justice Yates. The main question was whether or not the College had power to make such bye-laws and rules as they thought fit, and this was decided in their favour. But the words of the great Lord Mansfield in delivering judgment were remarkable, and left no doubt that he thought the College was insisting too rigidly on its rights. He cautioned the College against "narrowing their grounds of admission so much, that if even a Boerhaave should be resident here, he could not be admitted to their Fellowship." He said, "I would recommend the College to take the best advice in reviewing their statutes, and to attend to the design and intention of the Crown and Parliament in their institution. I see a source of great

[1] "A General View of the Establishment of Physic." Ferris, 195. "Letter to Lord Kenyon." Wells, 1795.

[2] "The Battle of the Wigs." Bonnell Thornton, 1778.

[3] For the full report of these cases, see "Burrows' Reports," Vols. IV and V, Rex *v.* Askew, and Rex *v.* R. C. P.

dispute and litigation in them as they now stand. There has not, it would seem, been due consideration had of the Charter, or legal advice in framing the bye-laws." As a result of Lord Mansfield's warning, the College passed a new bye-law by which Licentiates could be admitted to the examination for the Candidates for the Fellowship. But the new statute was all but inoperative, for, after having been proposed by a Fellow, the Licentiate was required to undergo three examinations, and the result of each examination, and the final admission as a Candidate for the Fellowship, depended on a vote of the majority of the Fellows present. So long, therefore, as the Fellows were almost unanimously opposed to the admission of Licentiates to their body there was little probability that a Licentiate would be allowed to come within the fold.

On May 16th, 1797, the whole subject was again raised in the Courts by Dr. Christopher Stanger, who applied to the Court for a mandamus commanding the College to show cause why he should not be examined for the position of Candidate for the Fellowship. The case was argued before Lord Kenyon, and the case for the College was in the able hands of Erskine. The composition of the Court was peculiar. Lord Kenyon had been for many years the standing counsel for the College, and was consulted regarding the drafting of the bye-laws after Lord Manfield's judgment. Of the other judges, Mr. Justice Lawrence was the son of a former President of the College, while Mr. Justice Grose and Mr. Justice Ashurst, the two remaining judges, were University men. Erskine told Dr. Stanger that he would much rather have pleaded his cause, but that counsel were like hackney coachmen, "First come, first served."[1] When the case opened Erskine at once cut the ground from under the feet of Stanger by citing the bye-law

[1] See Stanger's evidence before the Select Committee of the House of Commons, "Parliamentary Papers," 1834, p. 201.

passed after Lord Mansfield's admonition. He said, in effect, that Dr. Stanger could go before the College and be examined, and that the College could elect him to the Fellowship. Lord Kenyon agreed that the bye-law limiting the Fellows to the graduates in medicine of Oxford and Cambridge was bad, but since the College had passed a bye-law by which Licentiates could be examined for the position of Candidates for the Fellowship, he thought the bye-laws reasonable. He said, "If any one of the Fellows proposes Dr. Stanger, he goes to that tribunal which I hope and believe is the sanctuary of good faith and honour; . . . they are not bound to admit him, all they are bound to do is to examine him."[1]

After this case had been decided, Dr. William Wells determined to put the matter to the test in his own person, in order to see if the College would do that which they had expressed themselves as willing to do when before the Court, viz. to examine for the position of Candidate for the Fellowship any Licentiate who was proposed by a Fellow. Accordingly, Dr. David Pitcairn proposed, and Dr. Matthew Baillie seconded, that Dr. Wells should be allowed to present himself for examination. The College, however, refused the request, thereby deciding that the very bye-law on which they relied before the Court in May, 1797, was inoperative in September of the same year. Again Dr. Wells was proposed, but again various excuses were resorted to in order to prevent him from being examined. Then he desisted, for it was obvious that persistence was useless. Thus, William Charles Wells, Fellow of the Royal Society, Physician to St. Thomas's, and author of the "Essay on Dew," failed to become a Fellow of the College. His "Letter to Lord Kenyon," dealing with this episode, on account of its manliness, its spirit, its cogent reasoning, and its literary charm, should be read

[1] For the full report of this case, see "Law Reports," Rex *v.* College of Physicians, 1797.

almost as a model of what such specimens of composition should be. A few years later the President caused Dr. Wells to be asked if he still had any desire to become a Fellow, but to this he drily replied that he had none.[1]

This treatment meted out to Wells by the College had an unfavourable effect upon its reputation in after years. In 1834 a Select Committee of the House of Commons sat to enquire into the education and practice of various branches of the medical profession, and the case of Wells was made of capital importance by the Committee. Almost every witness was asked his opinion of the fitness of Wells to be a Fellow, and, to their credit, all, save one, admitted his great medical and scientific abilities as well as his unblemished character. Dr. William Macmichael, however, sought to depreciate the position of Wells in words which sound strange coming as they did from one who had been entrusted with the task of writing the "Lives of British Physicians." He said, "I am not aware that Dr. Wells was ever an eminent physician. He wrote some papers for the Royal Society on Dew, and was considered a clever man." After the Chairman had enumerated some eighteen papers by Wells, all dealing with medical subjects, he said, "There is one paper I do remember which is a very important one; that on rheumatism of the heart, all the others are such as the magazines and publications abound with at the present day. He is not the author of any great work." But the opinion of Dr. Macmichael is of no moment now, for inexorable Time has passed her judgment.[2]

[1] For a full account of this case see "A Letter to Lord Kenyon," Wells, 1799, and Stanger's "Justification," 1798.

[2] See "Parliamentary Papers," 1834, "Select Committee of House of Commons to enquire into medical education," and see page 39 for Macmichael's evidence. While pointing out that Wells was more scientific than medical Macmichael in the same breath instances Wollaston as an example of an eminent physician:—Wollaston who divorced

After the Parliamentary Committee had made a Report, the rule regarding the admission of Fellows was amended in such a way that a Licentiate could be admitted to the candidates' examination for the Fellowship without first becoming a Doctor of Medicine of either Oxford or Cambridge. The contest, therefore, which had lasted nearly a century, was ended, and the passions it had raised were stilled.

At the present day, the phases through which this contest passed have only an academic interest, and scarcely, perhaps, require notice except as forming part of the medical history under review. It may, however, be observed that out of this contest sprang those wise principles which govern at the present time the election of Fellows to the Royal College of Physicians.

THE MEDICAL PRESS

The development of the Medical Press during the age of George III has still to be considered. In those days no journals existed which dealt with the politics, the aims, and the aspirations of the medical profession. When a reformer arose his only method of disseminating his views was by means of "Letters," "Observations," and "Considerations." Most of these tracts, a splendid series of which exists in the library of the College of Physicians, are anonymous, and sometimes trivial, but to the student of the period they are often invaluable.[1] In the same way, apart from published books on medical subjects, many short mono-

himself entirely from medicine in his thirty-fourth year! The evidence given in this enquiry is invaluable from the point of view of the history of medicine. It may be remarked also that it contains the dramatic evidence of Clift regarding the destruction of Hunter's manuscripts by Sir Everard Home.

[1] Many of these compositions will be found, bound up with short monographs dealing with medical subjects, in the library of the College of Physicians. It is hardly possible to obtain a picture of bygone medical times without recourse to this species of medical literature.

graphs gave us the first introduction to new ideas and discoveries in medicine. During the reign many attempts were made to establish periodical medical publications. Some of them met with a fair share of success, and flourished for a number of years, but many survived only a short time. Dr. Dawson Williams has pointed out that the first English journal devoted to medicine appeared so long ago as 1684, but two numbers only were issued. This was followed in 1737 by " Medical Essays and Observations," published in Edinburgh, and continued until 1757. But with these two exceptions no medical journals existed until the reign of George III.

In 1757 " Medical Observations and Enquiries," promoted by a Society of Physicians, was established, and for many years enjoyed a considerable popularity. The next journal to appear was the " Medical Museum " in 1763, a volume devoted to " Select Cases and Experiments and Discoveries in Medicine and Pharmacy." The following year " Medical Essays and Observations " made its appearance, and was composed of abridged Memoirs of the Royal Academy of Sciences in Paris. After this in 1767 the " Medical Transactions " of the College of Physicians was begun, at the instigation of the elder Heberden. Six volumes of these " Transactions " were published, the last appearing in 1820. The " London Medical Journal " was founded in 1781 by Dr. Simmons, who was its first editor, and in 1791 it was continued as " Medical Facts and Observations." Dr. Simmons was also responsible for the " Medical Communications " which began in 1784 as the journal of the " Society for Promoting Medical Knowledge," but after two volumes were issued it ceased in 1790. Three volumes of the " Medical Spectator " were published between 1791 and 1796, and two of the " New London Medical Journal " in 1792–3. In 1793 the " Society for the Improvement of Medical and Chirurgical Knowledge " issued its first volume of Transactions, and at intervals two other volumes were published, the last appearing in 1812. They were all edited by Dr. Wells. The "Medical and Chirurgical Review" began its career in 1795, and continued until 1807. In 1799 the "Medical and Physical Journal" first appeared, and survived until 1833. The "London Medical Repository" was first published in 1814, and under various titles continued to appear until 1836. Besides these periodical publications, the Transactions of the Medical Society and of the Medico-Chirurgical Society were being issued from time to time. The list is a full one, and bears striking testimony to the great activity taking place in every branch of medicine during the closing years of the eighteenth century.[1]

It was not until 1823 that the "Lancet" appeared, and quickly enjoyed a wide popularity. The cause of its success was to be found in its powerful advocacy of medical reform, which was sadly needed, and in the great ability with which it was conducted. It not only appealed to the strictly medical mind, but also to the more progressive spirits in the profession, who relished its truculent tone towards existing medical authority. Its methods were sometimes questionable, but always undeniably clever, and when such matter as the incomparable "Intercepted Letters" by Wardrop appeared, although the medical world was convulsed with laughter, the fact cannot be denied that the good taste of such journalism was doubtful.[2]

[1] For a full list of all the medical periodicals see Appendix.

[2] See the earlier numbers of the "Lancet," and especially the issues of the years 1833–36 for the "Intercepted Letters." See also the "Life of Thomas Wakley," Sprigge, and "Autobiographical Reminiscences of the Medical Profession," Clarke.

CHAPTER II

THE ADVANCE OF MEDICAL KNOWLEDGE

In the previous chapter the general conditions under which medicine in England existed during the reign of George III were sketched. In this chapter it is proposed to give some account of the individual work of physicians of that period. For the purposes of this enquiry, the work of those physicians who contributed to the advancement of medical knowledge will be considered, and after that an estimate will be made of those who widened the boundaries of general science.

An investigation of this kind will not be without interest and profit, for it will bring us into closer contact with the personalities of those distinguished physicians who belonged to and influenced that medical age. But in appraising the work performed by these physicians little will be added to our stock of knowledge if we approach the subject in any captious spirit of criticism. We are often apt, in the light of later knowledge, to belittle the attempts of early investigators in the field of science. We see where they were blind; we can fill in the lacunæ in the chain of facts where they failed, and we forget that future ages may justly smile at our own puny efforts to unravel the mysteries of Nature.

The sources of information concerning the physicians of the age of George III are ample, but it must be confessed that most writers, in estimating the characters and life-work of their heroes, have adhered too closely, perhaps, to the dictum "de mortuis nil nisi bonum."

This is to be regretted, for however pleasing it may be to think that our profession has been content to deal kindly with the reputations of those who may have been rivals and competitors, the student prefers a pen-portrait with all the blemishes depicted. The medical writings of the age of George III can be studied, and a judgment passed concerning their merit, but for a knowledge of the personal characteristics of the physicians, recourse must be had to the "Gentleman's Magazine" the "Roll of the College," and the "Dictionary of National Biography." Some few of the more eminent physicians have attained to the dignity of a complete "Life," but for the large majority, these three sources of information just mentioned form, almost, our only guide to the lives and characters of the physicians of this period. Of first importance as contemporary evidence are the memoirs and obituary notices of physicians found scattered over the pages of that repository of biographical knowledge the "Gentleman's Magazine." These appreciations were written by men who were personally acquainted with the subjects of their memoirs, and it appears that trouble was taken to place the work of writing these notices in competent hands. Thus we know that the memoirs of David Pitcairn, George Fordyce, and Andrew Wilson proceeded from the able pen of Dr. Wells, and many others were undertaken by men equally qualified. The "Roll of the College" is a monument to the industry and ability of Dr. Munk, and is indispensable to the student of medical biography. Of course, in such a work, composed as it is of an enormous mass of facts and dates, absolute infallibility cannot be expected. But it may be stated with safety that few works of reference contain so few mistakes. Although the spirit in which Munk's biographies have been conceived may be somewhat lacking in fearless criticism, yet as a whole the work is admirable in point of style and justness.

Then the authors of "The Lives of British Physicians" have contributed much to the subject of medical biography, and the same may be said of Pettigrew and Aikin. They are all, however, open to the criticism that they make the subjects of their memoirs appear to be perfect paragons of private and professional virtue. Very valuable information concerning the Fellows and Licentiates of the College of Physicians during the first twenty years of the nineteenth century will be found in an anonymous work published in 1817, and entitled "A Picture of the College of Physicians." The biographies have considerable merit, and the author, whoever he may be, has exhibited a fairness and candour, in dealing with his subjects, worthy of praise. Finally, to complete the list of the sources of information respecting medical biography, mention must be made of the memoirs in the "Dictionary of National Biography." These may be regarded as the final pronouncements upon the lives and work of physicians of the past, founded on a study of all accessible authorities. The author of most of these memoirs is Dr. Norman Moore, and having said that it is only necessary to remark that the work could not have been placed in more capable hands and that the results are fully equal to the great reputation enjoyed by that writer of medical history.

Taken as a whole, the medical writings of the reign of George III exhibit a high degree of literary excellence, and often compare favourably with works of the same class at the present time. This is not a matter for surprise, for in those days a physician was generally possessed of considerable literary culture. At most Universities, and especially at Oxford and Cambridge, it was incumbent upon him to proceed to a degree in Arts, preparatory to the study of medicine, and the comprehensive nature of the instruction in Arts has already been described in the first chapter. While it may be true that the literary style of many medical works at this period savours too much of a rigid classical training, it is nevertheless a fact that many of them are almost models of clear exposition and elegant diction.

A review of medical work during the reign of George III, with special attention to its prominent exponents, may now be attempted. At the commencement of the reign, medicine was awakening from its long slumber, and the spirit of Harvey and Sydenham was beginning to reassert itself. The restricting and unsettling influence of the various "Systems" ceased to hamper the thoughts of physicians. They began to observe, to appeal to their own experience of disease, and to attempt to shape their views and practice in accordance with demonstrable facts. A race of pure clinicians arose, but as yet the fruits of the study of morbid anatomy, physiology, and chemistry were not within its reach. Still, using such means as they possessed, physicians became remarkably acute observers, and among them reckoned some of the greatest clinicians this country has produced.

An excellent idea of the scope of medicine taught during the first thirty years of the reign can be formed from a study of "The Elements of the Practice of Physic" by George Fordyce,[1] the celebrated physician of St. Thomas's Hospital. This book was, apparently, the student's text-book of those days, and enjoyed a wide popularity, passing through many editions. Fordyce was engaged for thirty years in lecturing on medicine at his house in Essex Street, Strand, and the "Elements of the Practice of Physic" may be taken as the substance of what he was accustomed to teach at these lectures. Some hundred pages of the book are devoted to the Natural History of the Human Body, or in modern terms, physiology. As might be

[1] "The Elements of the Practice of Physic," Geo. Fordyce. Fifth edition, 1784. First edition, 1770.

expected, at that early period in the history of physiology, the knowledge shown of this science was decidedly scanty, but nevertheless surprisingly free from gross errors.[1] The remaining part of the volume deals with the Symptoms, Distinctions, Prognostics, and Cure of Fevers and Inflammations, and under these headings is included the whole of the morbid conditions physicians were called upon to treat. In accordance with the doctrines regarding fevers prevalent at that time, little attempt is made to differentiate and classify the various forms, and the subject is treated of more or less as an entity. So also with inflammations; they were generalised so far as symptoms were concerned, and as to treatment, if they were sthenic, they called for revulsive measures, if asthenic, for tonics and stimulants. It is to be regretted that George Fordyce is remembered to-day more on account of his gastronomic feats at Dolly's Coffee House than for his long life of honest work in the cause of medicine. He was, indeed, a sagacious and scientific physician far in advance of his time, facts which rest on the assertion of so uncompromising a critic as Dr. Wells. He made no use of morbid anatomy as an aid to the practice of medicine, but he imparted to his pupils what was known of chemistry and physiology.[2]

Time does not permit of a detailed description of the characteristics of all the physicians who attained to eminence as clinicians during the first forty years of the reign, but some may be selected as typical of them all. The first to be mentioned is William Heberden the elder, and if terms partaking of exaggeration are used in speaking of that good and great man, the excuse

[1] Fordyce was evidently acquainted with the labours of Haller, Réaumur, and Spallanzani with reference to Digestion and Respiration.

[2] For an excellent account of the life and work of George Fordyce see "The Gentleman's Magazine" for June, 1802, from the pen of his friend and colleague W. C. Wells.

must be that the more one studies his life and work the less one finds to criticise and belittle. For Heberden is the great prototype of the modern clinician, the connecting link between Sydenham, and Bright, Addison and Watson. His "Commentaries," the book by which his name will be for ever perpetuated, was published after his death in 1801, but contains the results of his study and experience extending over sixty years. Remembering the time in which he lived, and the state of medical knowledge, it is truly a wonderful work, and must have acted on the medical world of that age like a refreshing breeze over arid and parched tracts. So sound is its doctrine, so cautious its treatment, and so endowed with excellent common sense, that much of it would require but little editing at the present day.[1] Here we find no fantastic theories, no appeal to metaphysical disquisitions, but simply the results of a close observance of signs and symptoms of disease at the bedside by an acute observer. Throughout the book Heberden strikes a note of honest pessimism, and when his knowledge and experience fail him, he is too great to be ashamed to own it. He shows also a righteous contempt for the vaunted specifics, and an adamantine refusal to accept anything incapable of proof, on whatsoever authority it might be stated. Almost in sorrow he closes his luminous pages with a humble apology for having been able to say so little that was valuable concerning a subject upon which he had been engaged for the whole of his long professional life. He even ventures the opinion that there was not much prospect of an advance in medical knowledge unless a prodigy, such as a medical Newton, should arise. Such was Heberden's book; the first clinical manual that had

[1] Yet Dr. Thomas Young, in his "Treatise on Consumption" has referred in slighting terms to the "Commentaries." Compare, however, this mine of observation and experience with Young's "Treatise," where, beyond a compilation of what others have said, Young has scarcely contributed a single observation of his own worth recording.

appeared. As a practical physician his reputation was already beyond the reach of criticism at the hands of his contemporaries, and with the "Commentaries" before them, successive ages of physicians will unreservedly endorse that verdict.[1]

Of Heberden's great qualities as a man and a scholar it is unnecessary to speak, for those, and his peculiarly endearing personality, have often been portrayed. Fortunate must have been the patient who came under his able and tender hands.

Many well-known eulogies of the character and work of Heberden are in print, but one noble appreciation, the finest of all, is wellnigh forgotten, and since it comes from the pen of Dr. Wells, who was no flatterer, it may be quoted. He says: "Dr. Heberden stands alone in his profession. No other person either in this or any other country has ever exercised the art of medicine with the same dignity, or has contributed so much to raise it in the estimation of mankind. Were I possessed of talents adequate to the undertaking, I should attempt to describe at full length the character of that illustrious man. In this attempt I should first mark his various and extensive learning, his modesty in the use of it, and his philosophical distrust of human opinions, however sanctioned by time or the authority of great names. I should then exhibit him in the exercise of his profession, without envy or jealousy, too proud to court employment, yet undervaluing his services after they were performed. Unwearied, even when a veteran in his art, in ascertaining the minutest circumstances of the sick who placed themselves under his care, taking nothing in their situation for granted that might be learned by enquiry, and trusting nothing

[1] Besides the "Commentaries," Heberden's Gulstonian Lectures exist in manuscript in the library of the College, and are delightful reading. The first three volumes of the "Transactions of the College" also contain many papers read by him.

of importance that concerned them to his memory. To demonstrate the greatness of his mind, I should next mention his repeatedly declining to accept those offices of honour and profit at the British Court, which are regarded by other physicians as objects of their highest ambitions, and are, therefore, sought by them with the utmost assiduity. I should afterwards take notice of his simple yet dignified manners, his piety to God, his love for his country, and his exemplary discharge of the duties of all private relations in which he stood to society, and I should conclude by observing that his whole life had been regulated by the most exquisite prudence. After my description was finished, I should think it proper to say that I had never been acquainted with Dr. Heberden, and consequently could neither be dazzled by the splendour of his virtues from approaching them too nearly, nor influenced in my opinion concerning them by benefits he had already conferred upon me; and that standing as he does on the verge of this state of existence ready to wing his flight to another glory, his ear must be closed to the voice of flattery, had he ever listened to that syren, or were I base enough to solicit her aid in the foolish expectation of receiving from him some future reward."[1]

Another of the great clinicians of this period was Sir George Baker, the distinguished President of the College of Physicians. But for one piece of epoch-making work he would have passed into history as an accomplished physician who enjoyed a more than usually large share of public favour, and whose classical attainments were of a higher order than those of any other physician, with the exception of Samuel Musgrave. Fortunately for posterity he investigated the cause of lead colic in Devonshire, and the result of this work

[1] The above eulogy occurs in "The Letter to Lord Kenyon," Wells, 1799.

is contained in a series of essays,[1] which may be justly quoted as models of inductive logic. It is not so much on the score of originality that Baker's essays are remarkable, for it had already been pointed out by Bouvart, Wall, and Zeller that lead held in solution in wines was the cause of plumbism at Poitou and other places. But it was the accurate reasoning contained in the essays that won for them such lasting renown. There is the irresistible marshalling of facts, the proof that the facts are indisputable, and the unerring deductions drawn therefrom which established for all time that the colic in Devonshire was produced by the presence of lead in the cyder. The chemical part of the enquiry was beyond the power of Sir George Baker, and this was placed in the hands of Dr. William Saunders of Guy's Hospital, and a portion of the credit for this undertaking is certainly due to him.

Now, this investigation concerning the nature of colic was first begun by Baker at the little village of Alphington in 1765, and is, therefore, one of the first attempts to grapple with a medical problem by means of the experimental method. No speculations were advanced, and the results of the experiments were the sole grounds for the deductions made.

A year previous to the work on Devonshire colic Baker had published an enquiry, scarcely less important, concerning the question of inoculation of small-pox.[2] Here, again, it is incontrovertible facts that he seeks. He gives an account of the method of performing inoculation, and the results as obtained by Dr. Pulteney in the town of Blandford, where thirteen

[1] The Essays appeared first in the "Transactions of the College," Vol. I, pp. 175–406, and were read in June, July, and August, 1767. Afterwards they were published in one volume entitled "Essays concerning the Cause of the Endemial Colic of Devonshire." 1767.

[2] "An Enquiry into the Results of a Method of Inoculating Small-Pox." 1766.

people died out of a total of 350 submitted to the operation.

Of Baker's merits as a practitioner we can only judge from the opinions formed by his contemporaries, and these were universally favourable. Indeed, few physicians were so respected, and not the least of his amiable qualities was his kindness shown to young physicians about to engage in practice in the metropolis.[1]

Other physicians during the last forty years of the eighteenth century attained great celebrity as clinicians, but since they have contributed little or nothing to medical literature it becomes difficult to assess their real merit. Contemporary evidence, however, is almost unanimous in according them high praise, and the estimates then formed must be accepted. Certainly no doubt can exist concerning the clinical abilities of Richard Warren, the two Pitcairns, Robert Gooch, and John Fothergill, and perhaps the same may be said of Henry Revell Reynolds and Sir Lucas Pepys. Coming much later, but belonging to the same class, was Sir Henry Halford, who may be regarded as almost the last of the old-time clinicians. He occupied for many years a conspicuous place in medicine, but great difficulty is encountered when the attempt is made to assign him his particular place. The enormous debt the College owes him for having been instrumental in placing the College on its present site, and for the admirable way in which he maintained its dignity, authority, and privileges for more than twenty years through most trying times, no one will for a moment deny. Nor will it be possible to contest the statement that his classical erudition was of a high order, and that he enjoyed a success in the practice of medicine beyond

[1] It should also be remembered to the credit of Sir George Baker that he was instrumental in finding funds to send Richard Porson to Cambridge. But for this act of kindness the world might have lacked the greatest Greek scholar.

most others.[1] But as to his claim to rank as an eminent exponent of the art of clinical medicine, it is quite possible, from such evidence as is available, to form hypotheses for and against that contention. The life and character of Halford have been presented to us from two distinct points of view. There is the admirable eulogy by Dr. Munk,[2] in which scarce an imperfection is admitted, save some slight hastiness of temper, and a tendency to carry the manners of the Court into private life. There are, also, the clever but unscrupulous "Intercepted Letters" of Wardrop,[3] in which every vulnerable part of Halford's character is exposed and ridiculed with a merciless satire and a biting sarcasm that reminds one of Voltaire in his most pungent mood. These represent the two sides of the picture, but are not of any great value as a contribution to historical accuracy. Halford may have been an excellent diagnostician, he certainly was an excellent prescriber, but in the midst of the pronounced advances that were being made in clinical methods he clung to the old traditions, and refused, to the end of his life, to have anything to do with the stethoscope. Perhaps the truth about Halford may be found to lurk in the fact that to a fair knowledge of medicine he united a shrewd and profound knowledge of mankind, and so succeeded where others failed.

But towards the end of the eighteenth century the existing order of clinical physicians, who depended for their medical acumen upon knowledge gained entirely

[1] It is often difficult to estimate the ability of physicians as classics. For instance, the Harveian Oration of Dr. John Latham has been described by Halford as a model of graceful Latin, but Dr. Wells, equally competent to judge, has described it as full of mistakes in grammar that would shame a schoolboy.

[2] "Life of Sir Henry Halford," Munk, 1895.

[3] See the "Lancet," 1834–37, under the heading "Intercepted Letters." Although undeniably clever they are a sad commentary on the bitter state of feeling in the profession of those days.

at the bedside, was beginning to be replaced by a race of men who enlisted the sciences of Chemistry, Anatomy, and Physiology for the purpose of elucidating the problems connected with disease. The pure clinician had reached a point beyond which it was almost impossible to advance. However much he might know concerning symptoms and their treatment, he could never attain to any real knowledge of disease without a study of the morbid anatomical and physiological conditions which caused it. His treatment, therefore, was entirely symptomatic, and he was inclined more and more to simplify and classify symptoms, while disregarding their true causes. His race was run, and he was compelled to make way for men with better equipment.

Why the sciences of Anatomy, Chemistry, and Physiology should have become dormant for nearly seventy years, after having given such remarkable promise at the end of the seventeenth century, it is most difficult to explain. But the fact remains that until Morgagni, Lavoisier, and Haller respectively rekindled the enthusiasm for Anatomy, Chemistry, and Physiology, nothing of great importance had been accomplished for more than half a century.[1] Morgagni revived Anatomy, Haller[2] Physiology, and Lavoisier gave the *coup de grâce* to the theory of Phlogiston which had cramped and starved Chemistry for nearly a hundred years. After the efforts of these three great men, the three sciences made rapid strides, and soon were in a position to lend their powerful aid to medicine.

Anatomy was the first science to be seriously applied to the service of practical medicine, and by its aid the

[1] Haller published his "Elementa Physiologiæ" in 1757. Lavoisier his "Sur la Nature du Principe" in 1775, and the English Translation of Morgagni's "De Sedibus et Causis Morborum" appeared in 1769.

[2] The work of Haller on Respiration, and of Réaumur and Spallanzani on Digestion contributed much to the practical application of Physiology to medicine.

medical vision was projected from the bedside to the post-mortem table. From time almost immemorial in the history of medicine human anatomy had been thoroughly taught, but mainly for the purpose of imparting a knowledge of the structure of the healthy human frame. But the possibilities of its practical application to the problems of disease were scarcely appreciated. This is somewhat strange when it is remembered that the best teachers at this time were physicians, among whom may be mentioned William Hunter, Frank Nicholls, James Douglas, James Parsons, Thomas Lawrence, and Matthew Baillie.

The desire to profit in medicine from knowledge gained by an examination of diseased parts on the post-mortem table received its first important stimulus in this country from the publication in 1769 of Dr. Alexander's translation of Morgagni's great work, "De Sedibus et Causis Morborum per Anatomen Indigatus."[1] In this work of the great Italian anatomist, for the first time anatomical knowledge was systematically devoted to the service of medicine. Not content with the mere description of the healthy parts of the human body, Morgagni broke with the somewhat inept tradition, and applied his knowledge to an anatomical investigation of diseased parts, in the endeavour to explain the symptoms and signs observed during the progress of disease. For all time he must be honoured as the first man to present a comprehensive picture of the possibilities of the study of morbid anatomy. But he had his limitations. More of an anatomist than a physician he was apt to pay more attention to the appearances observed after death than to those observed during life. He indicated the main characters of the disease, and laid bare the results obtained on the post-mortem table, but although the logical conclusion to be drawn appeared often to be irresistible, he hesitated—one had

[1] Morgagni published this book in 1761 when he was in his eightieth year.

almost said—feared to clinch the matter by a bold deduction.

Bîchat, the Napoleon of French medicine, carried on and advanced the study of morbid anatomy. What he accomplished in an all too brief life of thirty-one years does not belong to these lectures, but his name must be mentioned in connection with the movement.

But a greater than either Morgagni or Bîchat was about to arise in this country; great as a physician, great as a morbid anatomist, the father of medical pathology—the great figure of Matthew Baillie. With the blood of the Hunters in his veins, bred to anatomical pursuits under the immediate supervision of William Hunter, he stepped into the arena, as it were, in the nick of time. The older clinicians had completed their work, and it remained for Baillie to build a bridge over the gulf by means of which medicine could proceed to further perfection with the assistance of morbid anatomy. This he did by the publication in 1793 of his celebrated book "The Morbid Anatomy of some of the Most Important Parts of the Human Body." It was the first English treatise on Morbid Anatomy, and met with instantaneous success. In the preface to the first edition Baillie states in clear language the purpose of his work, which he summarises under four heads as follows: 1. "To explain the changes of structure arising from morbid actions." 2. "To distinguish between morbid changes which have been generally confounded." 3. "To detect diseased alterations in the organisation of parts which are but little, or not at all, known." 4. "From the observation of morbid structure, theories taken up hastily about disease will be occasionally corrected."

Such were the objects of Baillie's book, and from the date of its publication clinical medicine may be said to have obtained a new and extended charter eminently suited to its needs. The chief characteristics of the work are its admirable conciseness and its accurate observation. Unlike the overloaded volumes of Morgagni, the main important features of morbid anatomy, as described by Baillie, are not obscured by minute accounts of other trivial diseased conditions which played no part in the special morbid process under review. The wonderful plates, produced after the appearance of the book, even when viewed in the light of our present-day mature knowledge of morbid anatomy, are unimpeachable evidence of Baillie's unerring accuracy of observation. At that early stage of the study of the subject it could hardly be expected that any general principles regarding medical pathology would be enunciated, for Baillie was only building the foundations upon which future workers were to erect the superstructure of the science of pathology.

Great as was the effect of Baillie's book in this country, it met with almost greater success in Germany, where Professor Soemmering warmly embraced its doctrines and translated it into German. In England it soon began to exert its influence upon medical teaching, and in a little time every book dealing with medicine devoted an increasing space to the subject of morbid anatomy. Baillie, however, scarcely lived to see the full fruits of his pioneer work, and perhaps the importance of his innovation was hardly recognised by his immediate successors. But we, who live in the present age, can look back and detect in the work of Matthew Baillie the beginnings of the science of Pathology, which has ever since exercised such a profound influence upon the art of medicine. Indeed, we may almost assert that without Baillie the work of Abercrombie on the pathology of the brain and the intestinal canal, and of Bright on the kidneys, would have been postponed to a much later date. Few Fellows of this College have occupied a higher place.

At about the same time that Baillie was establishing the study of morbid anatomy, the sciences of Chemistry and Physiology were beginning to be seriously applied to the art of medicine. Much progress had been made in these sciences, and at the dawn of the nineteenth century they were so far developed that they were of the greatest service to medicine.

Previous to 1800 the science of Chemistry was in its cradle, and such teaching as was given was scanty and often erroneous. Still, long before that date the subject had received considerable attention by certain London physicians who were unwearied in their efforts to impart chemical knowledge. Dr. William Saunders, of Guy's Hospital, was one of the first to devote himself to the subject, and from 1766 onwards he lectured on Chemistry, and was justly regarded as one of its leading authorities among physicians. Others who worked in the same field were George Fordyce, William Babington, and Richard Powell. At about this period also the subject of Animal Chemistry began to attract the notice of chemists of eminence, and its study was greatly stimulated by Berzelius, who published his "View of the Progress and Present State of Animal Chemistry" early in the century.[1] But for some time the practical application of Physiological Chemistry to the proper understanding of diseased conditions received but scant notice by physicians, and was little understood. It was reserved for Dr. William Prout to be the first physician who brought to the aid of practical medicine a sound and comprehensive knowledge of Animal Chemistry. Prout's name stands high in the history of chemical science, and he forms one of the famous quartette of great scientists who adorned the medical profession towards the end of the reign of George III. But, unlike the other members of that quartette, Young, Wollaston,

[1] Young gives a translation of this work in his "Introduction to the Study of Medical Literature," 1813.

and Wells, Prout was distinguished for his practical ability as a physician, and his great attainments in science increased rather than diminished his reputation in this respect. In 1813 he began to lecture on Chemistry at his house in Southampton Street, and was honoured by having Sir Astley Cooper as one of his audience. Animal Chemistry engrossed his attention, and the first results of his researches appeared in 1821, when he published his book, " An Enquiry into the Nature and Treatment of Gravel, Calculus, and other Diseases of the Urinary Organs." It was the first treatise to deal with these diseases from a chemical standpoint, and marks the commencement of our knowledge of these conditions. In later editions of the work, Prout still further elaborated his views, and included the subject of digestion. Many fundamental truths concerning metabolism were first stated by Prout, among which may be mentioned the facts that urea was formed in the blood, and was merely excreted by the kidneys ; that the healthy stomach contained always a percentage of hydrochloric acid. Prout was also the first to enunciate the doctrine of " secondary assimilation," but unfortunately these views were, to a certain extent, purloined by Giessen and Justus von Liebig and given to the world under the high-sounding title of the " Metamorphoses of Tissues." But, always retiring and unobtrusive, Prout left it to others to point out that the theory had been promulgated by him several years before.

Although Prout may be regarded as the originator of the method of applying Chemical Physiology to the service of practical medicine, he was not the only worker in that sphere. Dr. A. J. Marcet a few years before had published an " Essay on the Chemical History and Medical Treatment of Calculus Disease," a book of the greatest merit, which did credit to his ability as a sound chemist. It is not, however, to be compared with the work of Prout, which went far beyond it in depth of insight and broadness of conception. Indeed, Prout did for Chemical Pathology what Baillie did for Morbid Anatomy, and must rank with him as a bold and sagacious innovator.

While these progressive movements were taking place in medicine and science, Robert Willan was pursuing his Dermatological investigations at the Public Dispensary in Carey Street. After many years' labour he gave to the world in 1798 his results in the shape of the first part of his great work on "Cutaneous Diseases." For the first time Willan placed the classification of diseases of the skin on an anatomical basis, from which proceeded all the developments in the knowledge of that subject. In order to appreciate the importance of Willan's work, one cannot do better than quote the admirable words of Dr. Pye-Smith, who says: "It is the great merit of Willan that he accurately described the anatomy of the morbid skin." His "orders," the "elementary lesions" of later dermatologists, are the alphabet of the subject, and correspond to the "physical signs" of disease of the lungs.[1]

Scarcely less important was the work of his pupil, Thomas Bateman, who still further advanced the subject of Dermatology. Besides being a pioneer in his special field Willan was a most accomplished clinician, and his abilities in this respect attracted to the Public Dispensary a large class of students, many of whom attained to the highest eminence. It is not often that teachers can claim as pupils a Bright, an Addison, a Marcet, and a Biett, but Willan and Bateman enjoyed that distinction. The Public Dispensary is still in existence, yet few know of it as the home of modern Dermatology under the able superintendence of the father of that branch of medicine, Robert Willan.

The subject of midwifery also made some progress

[1] See Fagge's "Principles of Medicine," first edition, Vol. II, p. 610.

during the reign, and was fostered by many able exponents of the art, among whom may be mentioned the names of Denman, W. Hunter, William Osborne, John Clarke, Hugh Ley, David Orme, and James Ford. Before 1739, apparently, no definite instruction was given in the subject in London, but in that year Smellie arrived in the metropolis and began a course of lectures. In the same year Sir Richard Manningham established a ward in the Westminster Infirmary for lying-in women, and this was the first attempt to find special accommodation for the study of midwifery. Soon after this, largely due, no doubt, to the influence of the teaching of Smellie, lying-in hospitals began to be erected, of which the first was the British Lying-in Hospital, founded in 1749 with William Hunter as its first physician. In 1769 Denman, who had been a pupil of Smellie, began a course of lectures in conjunction with William Osborne, and for fifteen years the majority of students attended these lectures. On October 6th, 1783, a greater importance was given to the status of the "man-midwife" by an Act of the College, which allowed those who practised midwifery to become Licentiates, and Thomas Denman was the first physician-accoucheur to receive that distinction.

For some time the introduction of medical men into the practice of midwifery was viewed by the public with much disfavour. Considerable commotion was occasioned in 1749 when Dr. Frank Nicholls gave lectures to men on the subject. The midwives and many of the laity were up in arms at this innovation which threatened their position, and Dr. Nicholls was under the necessity of explaining away his lectures by the publication in 1751 of his strange pamphlet entitled "The Petition of Unborn Babes to the Censors of the College." Even so late as 1830 a Society was founded, with Sir Anthony Carlisle as its president, for the avowed purpose of regaining for female midwives the position which had been usurped by the men. The Society was patronised by the Duchess of Kent and many other high-placed dames, some of whom had never been guilty of the impropriety of employing a physician-accoucheur. An extraordinary tract was written in 1830 by one M. Adams, entitled "Man-Midwifery Exposed," and scarcely on a much higher plane was the violent address of Sir Anthony Carlisle to His Majesty's Judges and Coroners, published in the "Times" on May 1st, 1830.

To judge from the views of experts in the subject, it would appear that Smellie must be regarded as the father of modern midwifery, while Hunter and Denman did more than others to improve its practice. After Smellie's day, however, it cannot be asserted that any great advance took place in Obstetrics during the reign of George III.

The work of those physicians who distinguished themselves in the realm of science during the reign under review must now be considered. There can be no doubt that the ranks of workers in Natural Science were largely recruited, at this period, from the medical profession, of which the College of Physicians contributed a goodly share. Indeed, a little reflection will show that it could not have been otherwise, for at this time the sciences of Chemistry, Anatomy, Physiology, and, to a certain extent, Botany were generally taught to those intending to become doctors. Until well after the commencement of the nineteenth century a man devoted to Natural Science could scarcely hope to maintain himself without the emolument and position that a degree in medicine secured. Many medical men, therefore, were engaged entirely in the study of science, and pursued the practice of the art of medicine with but little enthusiasm. It will not be necessary to mention the names of all those who applied themselves to scientific subjects, but attention will be paid to those physicians who were prominent in the cultivation of various branches of science. It has already been stated that the great names of Young, Wells, Wollaston, and Prout form a quartette of physicians who were superlatively great in science. The work of Prout has already been discussed, and attention will now be devoted to the activities of the other three.

In the van of all those physicians who have conferred honour upon our profession by reason of their mental attainments and scientific distinction stands the great name of Thomas Young, the glory of his or, it may be safely asserted, of any other medical age. It is almost impossible to realise the extent and depth of his mental capacity. Physics, Classics, Mathematics, Egyptology, Philology, Music, Biography, and Actuarial Science, he made them all his own, and to none of them did he devote himself without enriching them with his marvellous knowledge and power of application. Indeed, what Johnson wrote of Goldsmith might with equal truth be applied to Young: "Nihil tetigit quod non ornavit." If any man, however deeply and widely read, will take upon himself a study of the writings of Young, he will rise from his task with a chastened sense of his own inferiority, and will marvel at that comprehensive mind with its many and clean-cut facets, every one of which represented all that was known of a subject.

It is impossible for any but experts to follow him through all the particular branches of science and knowledge to which he devoted his powers. But Young has been fortunate in having a biographer who, with the exception of medicine, was qualified to speak with authority concerning all that the subject of his memoir had accomplished. It may, indeed, be doubted if any man of science has been so happily placed as Young in having his life-work described so ably by a natural philosopher who understood so well the difficulties of the subject. From the purely scientific side of Young's work, Dr. Peacock, his biographer, has given us as complete a picture as it is possible to exhibit, and his life of Young,[1] now sadly neglected, is exactly what a record of scientific work should be. It is an eminently just and critical estimate of his hero, unerring, precise, and able. Peacock's one failure was his inability to do justice to the medical side of Young's life. This is by far the weakest part of the book, and it is to be regretted that the chapter dealing with this subject was not entrusted to one more competent to criticise and pass judgment.

For a consideration of the work of Young, his life may be divided into three parts: 1. The time devoted to the equipment of his mind, 2. The time in which the results of that equipment were given out, and 3. His medical activities. Everything was to be expected of one who at the age of two years could read with fair fluency, and who at the age of four had read the Bible through twice. With Young there was never any hurry in the acquirement of knowledge; each subject in turn was taken up and deliberately exhausted before another was attempted. In this way, before he was twenty-one he was entitled to dispute with Porson and Parr concerning the niceties of Greek composition, and could hold his own in company on any subject. He was fortunate in having for a judicious adviser his uncle, Richard Brocklesby, who not only gave him excellent advice, but by a legacy of £10,000 and his house and its contents in Norfolk Street, Strand, relieved him of the necessity for drudging work in order to obtain a living. Edinburgh, Goettingin, and Cambridge claimed him as a student. In 1802, in his twenty-ninth year, he was appointed to deliver lectures on Natural Philosophy at the Royal Institution, and at about the same time he

[1] "Life of Thomas Young," George Peacock, 1855. See also Young's "Miscellaneous Works," 3 vols., 1855, edited by Peacock.

published his undulatory theory of light, by which his name will be for ever famous. It was not until 1816, however, that he really began to interest himself in Egyptology.

In all these branches of science Young was destined to meet with much opposition to his views, and much of his time was spent in answering opponents. Thus, his undulatory theory of light was attacked with ability but unscrupulousness by Brougham, in the "Edinburgh Review," and, largely owing to this attack, the scientific world, with the exception of Arago and Fresnel, hesitated for some years to accept his theory. In the domain of Egyptology Young met with even more opposition, and was doomed to see much of his work pilfered by others, of whom the chief offender was the great Champollion. But there can be no doubt now that Young can claim priority over Champollion in the discovery of phonetic hieroglyphics from the study of the Rosetta-stone.

The opinion may be advanced that Young himself was in part responsible for the persistent endeavours to rob him of the credit for his discoveries. In his writings he too often appears to resent the intrusion of others into the intellectual territory over which his regal mind held sway. He sometimes assumed a tone of superiority, as in the case of his criticism of Dr. Wells' "Essay on Dew,"[1] little calculated to soothe. His style was somewhat obscure, and not a little caustic. One almost fears to speak the words, but was Thomas Young entirely guiltless of envy and jealousy?

No dispute can arise concerning Young's position in science; but what can be said regarding his reputation as a physician? He devoted a large part of his life to the cultivation of the art of medicine, but he acquired no success in practice, and, whether he was waiting for patients in Welbeck Street or at Worthing, one has

[1] See "Miscellaneous Writings," Young. Vol. II, p. 414.

the feeling that he was engaged in an uncongenial occupation, and was chafing at the time thus spent, which might have been employed more profitably. In his two published works,[1] it is, indeed, a laborious Young who writes, but not the Young of science, with his brilliant deductions and wide conceptions. His "Treatise on Consumptive Diseases" is merely a compilation, and savours too much of having been written to attract those who visited Worthing for the benefit of that complaint.[2] The "Introduction to Medical Literature" displays a vast amount of learning, but in other respects is not remarkable. In fact, it must be admitted that the peculiar character of Young's mind was ill-suited to the study of the art of medicine. Great as he was in the exact sciences, he showed no adaptability when dealing with a subject so inexact as medicine.[3]

At the moral qualities of Young no one can cast a stone. In thought, in deed, in all the relations of life "immaculate" is the only word that can describe him. One almost seeks, as a relief from the invariable rectitude of his life, some human foible, but there is none. In admiration we gaze at the white marble figure of Young's intellect, perfect in symmetry, and without a flaw. Our only regret is that it lacks warmth.

But of all the great men of science produced in the reign of George III, Thomas Young rises above them all in mental stature and comprehensiveness of intellect, and the College of Physicians must ever account it a signal honour that it can number him amongst its Fellows.

1 "An Introduction to Medical Literature," Young, 1813. "A Treatise on Consumptive Diseases," Young, 1815.

2 It is a matter for astonishment that so great a physicist as Young should speak in slighting terms of Avenbrugger's "Method of Percussion." See p. 22 of the "Treatise."

3 One must not, however, forget that the late Dr. Dickinson gave Young praise, though qualified, as a physician. See "St. George's Hospital Gazette," 1893, p. 77.

Then there is the lonely but commanding figure of William Charles Wells, almost pathetic in its isolation. Success in the shapes of social fame and emolument was not for him. He began his career in London penniless, and after sixteen years of toil was unable to command an income of more than £307 from all sources. Ill-health clogged his steps; in his forty-third year he was seized with a slight stroke, and henceforth for him it was a grim fight against time to finish the work he had designed. But in spite of these disadvantages he laboured on bravely in his humble lodging in Serjeant's Inn, scarcely known to any but five close friends, and when his work was accomplished he desired only the modest epitaph that "he had tried to extend the boundaries of knowledge." Shrewd judges of mankind, such as Brodie, described Wells as one of the most remarkable intellects of the age, but his peculiar temperament and somewhat cold, scientific type of mind did not lend themselves to the showy mental exploits so beloved by the multitude. As evidence, however, of his commanding abilities and personal character it will surely be sufficient to state that he was loved and respected by Matthew Baillie, David Pitcairn, and David Hume.

In the sphere of Natural Philosophy the name of Wells will be for ever honoured. It was his good fortune to investigate and establish the laws which govern the formation of moisture in the air, and although physical chemistry has advanced in all directions, the fundamental principles enunciated by him have never been seriously challenged. For this work Wells was awarded the Rumford medal in 1814, and since then his name has been inseparably connected with the subject.

What was the nature of this experimental work of Wells concerning dew? Previous to his work it had been supposed, since the days of Aristotle, that dew was formed in the lower atmosphere in consequence of its moisture being condensed by means of cold, and that in its formation cold was produced. This was the accepted view of Six, Wilson, Prevost, and Wells himself, after various experiments. On mature reflection, however, Wells became doubtful of the accuracy of this view, and accordingly determined to conduct a series of experiments with the object of testing his theories. These experiments were carried out in the garden of Mr. James Dunsmure, the merchant friend of Wells, who lived in Surrey, three miles from Blackfriar's Bridge, and therefore conveniently close for Wells, whose house was in Serjeants' Inn. To this country house Wells betook himself late in the afternoons, and, with varying intervals, caused by ill-health, prosecuted his experimental work during the nights, returning in the early morning to his house for the day's work. In his published "Essay on Dew"[1] he pays an affectionate tribute to his friend Dunsmure for allowing him to use his garden "at considerable inconvenience to the members of the family." Wells also conducted experiments in Lincoln's Inn Fields when increasing infirmity rendered it impossible for him to go into the country. Dunsmure's garden cannot now be located, but Lincoln's Inn Gardens still remain, and are surely hallowed by that association with Wells and his work.

For his experiments Wells used pieces of wool of known weight, and these he weighed again after they had absorbed the dew in various situations and under varying conditions of atmosphere. He thus became acquainted with the laws which govern the deposition of dew. For instance, he found that the exclusion of the sky from the wool diminished the quantity of dew formed, that more was deposited on wool when on grass than when placed on gravel, mould, bright metals, or when suspended in the air. Having obtained these data,

[1] "An Essay on Dew," Wells, 1814.

he then investigated the part cold played in the formation of dew, and at this stage his original discovery was made. He found, as others had done before, that the temperature of the ground was higher than that of the air above, that passing clouds caused a rise of temperature, and, what was of the utmost importance, that certain substances placed on the ground took on a lower temperature than the ground itself. From these facts he deduced his theory that "Dew is the production of a preceding cold in the substances upon which it appears." He also established the fact that the formation of water from the atmosphere actually produces heat. All this was contrary to the view, hitherto accepted, that dew was formed by the cold of the night, and that in its formation cold was produced.

Such was the work of Wells. It is a melancholy picture, this last effort of his, feverishly labouring to finish his experiments, with water-logged legs, and the agony of cardiac asthma ever present; spending nights in Dunsmure's garden which should have been devoted to repose, and then hurrying back to Town in the early morning to write down his results lest death should claim him ere his task was completed. Surely few scientific workers have battled so bravely with adverse conditions.

The medical work of Wells has not, perhaps, received the consideration it deserves, but a study of it will confirm the opinion that he was a highly original physician. His chief claim to distinction in this sphere rests on the papers he communicated to the Society for the Improvement of Medical and Chirurgical Knowledge, in which he dealt with the occurrence of albumen in cases of dropsy. His first paper, read on November 4th, 1806,[1] related only to cases of dropsy following scarlet fever. This phenomenon had been observed by Plenck, of Vienna, Cruikshank, and Berserius long

[1] See Vol. III, p. 167.

before, but it was Wells who noticed that blood and albumen were present in the urine in these cases. He also established the fact that the dropsy occurred in the upper parts of the body, and described without, however, giving them a name, the uræmic seizures to which such cases are liable. He found evidences of inflammation present in all the abdominal organs, including the kidneys, and inferred that the process was essentially inflammatory in origin.

On June 4th, 1811, he read another paper before the same Society,[1] which is marked by his accustomed care and skill in scientific investigation. Here he pointed out that albumen was to be found in cases of dropsy other than scarlatinal, and drew a distinction between hydrothorax, ascites, and dropsy of the skin, in that the two former, if primary, did not have albumen in the urine. This was the first attempt to differentiate between the various forms of dropsy. The point was used with great advantage by Blackall,[2] who, writing two years later, still further elaborated it, but the merit of pointing it out belongs to Wells alone. In support of his contentions Wells quoted two post-mortem examinations, in one of which "the kidneys were much harder than they usually are, and the cortical parts were thickened," while in the other he says "the kidneys were larger and softer, and on the outside were several vesicles." He gave the credit of the discovery of albumen to Cruikshank, who mentioned it in 1798, but points out that he had discovered it independently in 1799. Wells had, therefore, established the fact of albumen in dropsy. He had differentiated the forms of dropsy in which albumen is found. He had even indicated that the kidneys were diseased, but he failed to point out the causal relation-

[1] See Vol. III, p. 194.

[2] "Observations on the Nature and Cure of Dropsies," Blackall, 1813.

ship between the two. This momentous clinical fact had to await the advent of Richard Bright, but it was Wells who prepared the ground.

To complete the consideration of the work of Wells it must be remembered that Darwin himself, in his historical introduction to the "Origin of Species," gives to Wells the credit of having been the first to enunciate the principle of natural selection, in a paper read before the Royal Society in 1813. Surely this is the most precious jewel in his scientific crown.

Wells was an excellent classic, and wrote Latin with ease and correctness. In the literature of his own tongue he was widely read, and as a writer of vigorous and even elegant English it may be doubted whether he had a superior in the medical profession. While on his death-bed he dictated an autobiography [1] to his friend Mr. Patrick which is worthy of perusal as an honest and fearless estimation of his character and work. Altogether, Wells was one of the great men of our profession during the reign of George III; a man of great scientific ability, with a lofty conception of duty, and with an adherence to truth which never swerved.

William Hyde Wollaston was so little associated with the practice of medicine that his work can scarcely be considered from that point of view. Very early in his career he definitely severed his connection with medicine, owing, it is said, to his unsuccessful application for the post of physician to St. George's, and henceforth devoted himself entirely to science. Some of his scientific work, however, related to problems in medicine, and in this field he initiated enquiry which led to important results. He was one of the first to study the composition of calculi, and other abnormal constituents of the urine; work which, no doubt, paved the way for

[1] This interesting autobiographical sketch is prefixed to the posthumous edition of the "Works of Dr. Wells," issued in 1818.

the further extension of the subject by Prout and Marcet. He also explained the phenomenon of hemianopia, and demonstrated the partial decussation of the fibres in the optic commisure. But, with these exceptions, the whole of the scientific work of Wollaston belonged to Physics, Chemistry, and Metallurgy. He discovered Rhodium and Palladium, and devised a process for rendering Platinum malleable. He was the first to see the dark lines in the spectrum, since known under the name of Fraunhofer's Lines, but failed to appreciate their true significance. As a point of peculiar interest at the present time, it may be mentioned that Wollaston invented the periscope, an instrument so frequently in our thoughts to-day.

Excessively cautious, fearing to advance by bold deductions, Wollaston constantly allowed others to reap where he had sown. In this way he lost his claim to be one of the first sponsors of the Atomic Theory, and the judgment passed on him by Dr. Peacock, to the effect that on account of these failings his name is unconnected with great epochal advances is eminently correct.[1] It should, however, be mentioned that Wollaston shares with Sir Hans Sloane and Sir John Pringle the honour of being one of the three Fellows of the College who have reached the dignity of the Presidential chair of the Royal Society.

We have now completed the sketch of the progress made in medical knowledge during the reign of George III. We have seen that soon after the beginning of the reign a distinct revival of activity in its study became evident. We have shown that, at first, the revival manifested itself in an increase of clinical knowledge gained almost entirely from observation of symptoms during illness. We have pointed out the manner in which the obstacles to the advance of clinical medicine

[1] See "Life of Thomas Young," by Geo. Peacock, 1855, p. 469, quoted also by Munk, "Roll of the College."

were surmounted by the application of the sciences of pathology, physiology, and chemistry, which, towards the end of the eighteenth century, had been placed upon a sound foundation. We have also devoted space to the consideration of those physicians whose activities were mainly scientific. In all this the main features of the spirit of the eighteenth century, which laboured unceasingly for the emancipation of the human intellect, for freedom of thought, and for enquiry on scientific lines, can be clearly observed. We owe to the physicians of the age of George III an immense debt for the excellent foundations they built, often with rough and improvised tools. Like the Georgian architecture, the Georgian silver, and the Georgian glass, they were large and solid, and were fashioned to stand the test of time. Men of the stamp of Hunter, Baillie, Prout, and Willan flung open the portals of medical science, through which their descendants have passed to realms of spacious and accurate knowledge.

CHAPTER III

MEDICINE IN RELATION TO THE STATE

Lunacy—Prisons—Vaccination—Public Health—The Army Medical Service—The Walcheren Expedition.

In order to complete the review of the state of medicine in England during the reign of George III, it will be necessary to consider at some length the large subject of medicine in relation to the State at that period. This will involve an enquiry concerning the principles of medical treatment of the insane, prisoners, and paupers; the rise and effects of vaccination; the inception of sanitary science, and the development of the medical services in the Navy and Army. The study of these special branches of medicine is important, for during the reign of George III the principles which govern their practice at the present day were formulated and instituted. Since that time, although many changes in detail have occurred, the framework built in those days has undergone but little alteration.

LUNACY AND MADHOUSES

In no department of medicine during the reign of George III was the spirit of improvement at a lower ebb than in that of the care and treatment of the insane. It appeared to be the settled conviction of alienists that the principles of the treatment of mad people were satisfied by locking them up securely and by curbing their obliquities by means of barbarous coercion, and other cruel repressive measures. Men at the head of this particular branch of medicine seemed to be content with these methods. For instance, Dr. Monro, the able superintendent of Bethlem, when before the House of Commons Committee, apparently regarded it as nothing unusual that a patient under his care at Bethlem had been for nine years with iron collars round his neck and waist, and fettered to the wall with heavy chains. His only justification for such a proceeding was that the patient was "one of the most mischievous and ferocious lunatics he had ever known."[1] But while the majority of alienists held these views an exception must be made in the case of Dr. Battie, who was physician to St. Luke's. In this institution, under his influence, coercion had always been tempered with some show of kindness, and Dr. Rawes, the late superintendent, has said that many of the rules and regulations framed by Battie 150 years ago require but little alteration at the present day.

To appreciate the whole squalid story of the manner in which the insane were cared for and treated in the reign of George III, it is necessary to read the evidence given before the Committee of the House of Commons in the years 1813–15. That evidence recounts such acts of cruelty and callous negligence that go far beyond the wildest flights of the imagination of the uninstructed writer of romance. These poor creatures were beaten, starved, and manacled for acts over which they had no control. For months at a time they were cast into filthy dungeons with no light or clothing, and with only excrement-sodden straw on which to lie. Amputations of the fingers and toes, on account of frost-bite, were by no means uncommon. The practice of feeding by force was often resorted to, not on account of refusal to take food, but as a punishment, and from the barbarous

[1] Nearly the whole of this account of the condition of lunatics has been taken from the evidence given before the House of Commons Committee during the years 1813, 14, and 15. See "Parliamentary Papers" under the heading "Madhouses."

method employed death from suffocation was often the result. It rested with the keepers of the madhouse to decide whether an enquiry before a coroner should take place in case of sudden death, and it was given in evidence that the jurors were often chosen by the keeper. Nearly all the madhouses in London, of which there were thirty-seven, were managed by people who had been keepers in similar institutions, and an apothecary was called in to attend those who were sick. Rank of patients procured no amelioration of their wretched state. A captain of the Guards was beaten by a keeper so severely that he died, and a colonel was confined in a cell for several months naked, with nothing but dirty straw for a bed. A smith in London Wall prospered in his business on account of his special skill in forging fetters and chains for the hapless lunatic. If the madman made a noise he was gagged. In many places rats swarmed, and one witness swore that he had seen a patient call by name from their holes forty rats that she had tamed. Rat bites were common, and vermin infested the cells. No attempt at medical treatment of the insane was made, and the physicians appointed to inspect these places did their work in the most perfunctory manner. Violent patients were bled until they became exhausted, and acts of immorality sometimes took place between the keepers and the female patients. In fact, when one reads the evidence before this Committee of the revelations of Mrs. Humieres, of the iniquities of Rambaud and Dowding, and of the horrors of "Bella's Hole," a feeling of unreality seizes the mind.

It is sad to have to record the fact that it was not from the medical profession that any suggestion of improvement came, but from several noble-minded legislators, of whom the names of Townshend, Rose, Lord Robert Seymour, and Lord Binning will ever be remembered. The first attempt at legislation came in

February, 1763, when Mr. Townshend presented to the House of Commons a report on the condition of madhouses.[1] From this report it was evident that the condition of these places was very bad, and that the lunatics were admitted to them in a very loose manner. No real inspection ever took place, and the keepers were in the habit of admitting patients on the simple request of their relatives. In many instances those admitted were perfectly sane, and were incarcerated for nefarious purposes. As a result, regulations were framed for the better conduct of the madhouses, but in 1773 Mr. Townshend again brought up the subject, and placed the report of 1763 before the House. A bill was then introduced and passed in the following year, by which the inspection of madhouses was placed in the hands of visitors appointed by the College of Physicians. By this Act, five Commissioners were to be elected annually by the College, three of whom, with a secretary, were to be required to visit once a year every madhouse in London and seven miles around, and for this work they were to receive a guinea each for every madhouse visited. The powers of the Commissioners were, however, limited, for although they were able to withdraw a licence, the magistrates had no power to refuse a regrant, provided sufficient security was forthcoming.

Under this arrangement the condition of madhouses showed no tendency to improve, and it must be admitted that the Commissioners expended little time and trouble in the performance of their duties.[2] Very soon a strong feeling arose that the treatment of lunatics was a reproach to the country, and that the time was

[1] For a full account of this Report see "Parliamentary History," Vol. XV. (Report *re* Madhouses, 1763.)

[2] It was given in evidence before the Committee, that a Commissioner visited a house in Hoxton and claimed to have examined 405 inmates in two and a half hours.

ripe for a movement in the direction of the amelioration of their unhappy condition. There were several reasons for this change of opinion. The Draconian age of legislation was passing away; the teaching of Pinel, which was the antithesis of force in the treatment of the insane, was beginning to be known in England, and, under the influence of the Tukes, the Retreat at York had been opened, where methods of kindness and persuasion took the place of cruelty and repression. Finally, to these causes must be added the repeated attacks of insanity from which George III himself suffered, and which impressed the subject upon the minds of legislators. The result of these conditions was the Select Committee of the House of Commons in 1813, to which reference has already been made. On June 17th, 1816, a bill was promoted, by which it was intended to repeal the Act of 1774 and to appoint eight Commissioners, under the jurisdiction of the Home Secretary, who, with the assistance of two magistrates, were to be responsible for the care of all madhouses.[1] This bill, however, failed to become law, and it was not until some years later that legal effect was given to the findings of the Select Committee. But the conscience of the nation had been awakened, and afterwards, largely owing to the great work of Connolly, the foul stain of our horrible treatment of the insane was removed from the annals of the country.

The physicians chiefly responsible for the care of lunatics during the reign of George III were William Battie, Thomas Brooke, Samuel Foart Simmons, and A. R. Sutherland, all of whom were physicians to St. Luke's. Three generations of the family of Monro,

[1] See an interesting speech on June 17th, 1816, by Lord Robert Seymour regarding the condition of madhouses. Hansard, 1816. Also "The Pamphleteer," Vol. VI, for the findings of the Committee on Madhouses. The whole subject, however, should be read in the evidence published in "Parliamentary Papers" Select Committee of House of Commons on Madhouses, 1813–16.

viz. James, Thomas, and Edward, held sway at Bethlem, and to these must be added Dr. Francis Willis, D.D. and M.D., at one time vicar at Wapping, but famous as the physician in attendance upon the King. In addition to occupying these positions, they were all interested in private houses for the insane, out of which they accumulated large fortunes. They do not, however, appear to have contributed much to the advancement of their speciality.

PRISONS

The sanitary condition of prisons was scarcely less deplorable than that of madhouses during the reign of George III, and was hardly considered to be a subject requiring reform by even the most enlightened publicists. Nor will this attitude cause astonishment when it is remembered that legislation occupied itself solely with punishment for misdeeds, and took no account of prevention of crime by elevating the moral tone of the criminal. The medical care of prisons was in the hands of apothecaries. No regular attendance was required, and it was left to the governor of the prison to determine whether the visit of the apothecary was desirable.[1] Even in the cases of the large debtor prisons, the "King's Bench," the "Marshalsea," and the "Fleet," no medical man was appointed, and the inmates were dependent upon the good offices of some medical debtor prisoner for treatment when sick. The insanitary condition of these prisons was terrible, and such hotbeds of vice and disease were they that the assistant-master of the "Fleet," in his evidence before the Parliamentary Committee, shamelessly described his prison as the largest brothel in London.[2] The jails

[1] See "History of Medicine," John Mason Good, 1796.

[2] See "Report of the Parliamentary Committee on the 'King's Bench,' 'Marshalsea,' and 'Fleet Prisons,'" 1814. The evidence before this Committee is also published in "The Pamphleteer," Vol. VI.

were veritable forcing-houses for typhus and other contagious complaints, and many of the great epidemics could be traced to these places. The work of John Howard contributed much to the improvement of sanitary conditions in the prisons, but for a long time little real progress was made. The Poor Law, also, was administered with scarcely any regard for the medical care of the paupers, whose lot was most unfortunate. They were left to the care of the "Master" of the workhouse, and, when ill, it was his province to decide whether medical aid was necessary.

VACCINATION

In 1798 Edward Jenner published his "Enquiry into the Causes and Effects of Variolæ Vaccinæ," and thus established his claim to be the first to advocate vaccination as a preventive of small-pox. He was not the first, however, to practise this method, for Benjamin Jesty, a farmer in Dorset, had previously, in 1774, vaccinated some of the members of his family. It is not, however, proposed to proceed here upon the well-beaten track of the history of the discovery of vaccination by Edward Jenner. That subject has been already exhausted by many able authorities, and especially by Professor Crookshank, whose notable book is in truth the last word on the question.[1] The struggle for the supremacy of vaccination which took place in the early years of its history may, however, be briefly described.

In its inception, vaccination, like every other revolutionary medical advance, was compelled to fight for its existence. For eighty years inoculation had been the recognised method for protection from small-pox, and in the hands of the Suttons and Dimsdale it had become

[1] "History and Pathology of Vaccination," 2 vols. Crookshank, 1889. This work is valuable to the student on account of the reprints of many papers connected with the early history of vaccination.

as safe in its operation as such a dangerous procedure could be. Vaccination, on the other hand, was new; its exact mode of action was imperfectly understood, and it was necessary to rid it of avoidable accidents before it could be accepted as superior to inoculation. It has been the custom to visit with unusual censure the action of Benjamin Moseley, William Rowley, George Lipscombe, John Birch,[1] and others in their opposition to vaccination. As reactionaries, no doubt, they merited a measure of blame, but the rancour displayed by them was repaid with interest by the supporters of the newer method, and it cannot be denied that they had some ground for their opposition. But in no long time vaccination triumphed over all obstacles, the weaker supports of its theory were replaced, proof of its efficacy became overwhelming, and one of the richest blessings was conferred upon suffering mankind.

The great name of Jenner deservedly overshadows all others connected with the movement, and we are apt to forget the meritorious labours of his associates. George Pearson and William Woodville[2] at once championed the new method, and submitted it to extensive tests. Woodville, on account of the position he held of physician to the small-pox hospital, was able to conduct his experiments under most favourable circumstances, and it may be doubted whether vaccination would have made such rapid progress without his valuable co-operation.

[1] In order to appreciate the position of the Georgian anti-vaccinationists, the following tracts should be read: "Treatise on Lues Bovilla," B. Moseley, 1805. "Cow-Pox Inoculation," William Rowley, 1805. "Manual of Inoculation," George Lipscombe, 1806. "Reasons for Objecting to Vaccination," John Birch, 1806. These tracts, of course, seem puerile at the present day, but were formidable in the early years of the eighteenth century.

[2] See "An Enquiry Concerning the History of Cow-Pox," George Pearson, 1798. "Reports of a Series of Inoculations for the Variolæ Vacinæ or Cow-Pox," Woodville, 1799.

PUBLIC HEALTH

During the greater part of the reign of George III, such efforts as were directed towards the improvement of public health were made by private individuals, for no authority existed for this purpose. When epidemics of unusual severity took place, the matter was often referred to the College or to physicians who were authorities on the subject. A report was then drawn up and appropriate measures were instituted to combat the condition. Several physicians, however, made the incidence of disease in the metropolis their especial study, among whom must be mentioned the names of Heberden, Reid, Willan, Blane, and Bateman. Willan may be said to have been the first physician to make a systematic study of the health conditions of London, and in 1796 he began his "Monthly Reports on the Diseases of London," which were originally published in the "Monthly Magazine," but were afterwards collected in one volume in 1800. In 1805 Pitt made the first attempt to establish State control of public health when he brought into being his "Board of Health," but after a brief existence of a few months it was abolished in the following year. Some years later another Board was set up, and on this the College of Physicians was well represented. The subject of Public Health, however, was not seriously considered by the State until after the work of Southwood Smith and George Birkbeck had awakened the conscience of the nation, but the efforts of these two great pioneers belong to a later period, and do not properly fall within the scope of these chapters.

THE ARMY MEDICAL SERVICE

Vast changes took place in the Army Medical Service during the reign of George III, and it becomes important to study them with attention, for they often afford an explanation of the various stages through which the service passed until its permanent foundations were laid.

The early history of the Army Medical Service is somewhat obscure and difficult to follow with any accuracy, but the germ of the system is to be found, at any rate so far as regards its control, in the practice which obtained from early times of appointing a physician, and sometimes a surgeon, to accompany the monarch or the commander-in-chief when he went to the war.[1] Naturally, they were appealed to by the commander in any medical difficulty that arose, and soon, in addition to being responsible for the health of the head of the Army, they were entrusted with the care of the health of the Army as well. During the Civil War a serious attempt appears to have been made to place the medical department of the Army under proper supervision, and to this end the Parliament ordered three physicians, one of whom was Paul de Laune, to be attached to the Army under the command of the Earl of Essex. The commission lists of the Cavaliers and the Roundheads[2] also show that to each regiment a regular surgeon was attached. In 1649 a further step was taken, and Jonathan Goddard was appointed by Cromwell to the post of "First Physician" to the Army. In this capacity Goddard accompanied Cromwell to Scotland and Ireland, where he was succeeded by Sir William Petty in 1752.[3] The position of a single medical head in supreme authority over medical matters in the Army was thus established, and in much the same way a surgeon came to exercise

[1] Thomas Muffett, a Fellow of the College of Physicians was probably the first to be appointed Physician to an Army, when he was attached to the Expedition to Normandy, under the Earl of Essex in 1591.

[2] See Peacock's "Lists of the Cavaliers and the Roundheads."

[3] See "Munk's Roll," Vol. I, under Goddard, Petty, and De Laune. Also Dalton's "English Army Lists," and Johnstone's "Roll of the Army Medical Service."

supervision over surgeons and their duties. At first, these chief physicians and surgeons held their appointments only during the progress of a war, but in 1660, when a standing army was authorised, a Physician-General and a Surgeon-General were appointed, who exercised authority continuously during peace and war. The first Physician-General to be appointed was Thomas Laurence in 1685, and the first Surgeon-General was John Knight, appointed in 1664. Physicians and Surgeons-General were also appointed for Scotland and Ireland, and from 1660 until 1756 little material change was made in the method of government of the medical department in the Army.

According to Richard Brocklesby,[1] the first attempt to form an Army Medical Board of Control was made in 1756 by the Duke of Cumberland, who desired Viscount Barrington, Secretary of State at War, to establish a Hospital Board for the Army. This Board was composed of the Physician-General, the Surgeon-General, the physicians to hospitals, the Principal Surgeon of Hospitals, and the Purveyor-General, who were ordered to consult together concerning hospital matters. This Board recommended that the physicians should examine, superintend, and control the hospital mates, but that the surgeons should be allowed to nominate mates for their own department. Much was expected from the deliberations of the Board, and had time allowed, no doubt, many salutary reforms would have been instituted. But the career of the Board was suddenly cut short by the outbreak of war, when the physicians to hospitals and most of the surgeons were sent abroad, and the Principal Hospital Surgeon, after having been appointed Inspector of Regimental Infirmaries, gradually assumed all the functions of the

[1] See "Economical and Medical Observations from 1758 to 1762, Tending to the Improvement of Military Hospitals," Brocklesby, 1764, p. 31.

Board. He appointed all the hospital mates and accepted the examination at the Surgeon's Hall as a test of fitness. The Board, therefore, virtually ceased to exist, and was not revived again until 1793.

During the early part of the reign of George III, the post of Physician-General was held successively by Sir Edward Wilmot and Sir Clifton Wintringham, who owed their appointments respectively to George II and the Duke of Cumberland. The combined posts of Surgeon-General and Inspector of Regimental Infirmaries was held, first by Mr. Adair, and afterwards by the great John Hunter.[1] On Hunter's death in 1793 the two appointments held by him were separated, and two of his surgical colleagues at St. George's, Mr. Gunning and Thomas Keate, were appointed respectively Surgeon-General and Inspector of Regimental Infirmaries. At this time it was apparently felt that the supreme direction of medical matters in the Army required some co-ordination, for Wintringham was in his eighty-third year, and incapacitated by infirmities from attending to business. Gunning and Keate were accordingly instructed to consult together regarding all Army medical affairs, including the appointment of physicians, surgeons, and hospital mates. In this manner the Army Medical Board was reconstituted. On January 15th, 1794, after the death of Wintringham, Sir Lucas Pepys was appointed Physician-General as a reward for services rendered to the King during his illness in 1789. Pepys had no special knowledge of the conditions and requirements of the Army Medical Service. He had never served in the Army, and much will be said hereafter concerning his influence during the fifteen years he occupied this position. From 1794 to 1798 the three members of the Board performed

[1] Sir Edward Wilmot held this position from 1740 to 1787, and Sir Clifton Wintringham from 1787 to 1794. Hunter held his posts for three years, although he had been Deputy Surgeon-General for several years.

their functions in a collective capacity, and although they each had their special departments, the Board as a whole was responsible to the Commander-in-Chief for the acts of each member.

In 1798 Gunning died, and his position of Surgeon-General was assumed by Keate, while Mr. Rush was appointed Inspector of Regimental Infirmaries in place of Keate. Rush died in 1801, and was succeeded by Francis Knight, that appointment being now styled Inspector-General of Hospitals. On March 12th, 1798, a new order regarding the Army Medical Board was issued by the Commander-in-Chief, by which many of its collective functions were abrogated, and each member was made, more or less, supreme in his own department.

The precise functions of each member of the Board, as it now existed, will be found in the "Report of the Commissioners for Military Enquiry for 1808,"[1] and in the evidence given by the members of the Board before the House of Commons in 1810, regarding the Walcheren Expedition.[2] Surely it is impossible to imagine a more clumsy and impossible arrangement. Even after a patient study of these documents it is a most difficult matter to determine the functions of the Board in either its individual or collective capacity. The position, so far as can be ascertained, was as follows: Collectively the Board was supposed to meet if questions were submitted to it. It was to obey orders, but it was no part of its business to make representations, and when it did meet the Physician-General took the chair. In their individual capacities the members were assigned special duties, but the conduct

[1] In this account of the Army Medical Board, the information found in the evidence given before the Commissioners for Military Enquiry in 1808 has been used. The Fifth Report of the Commissioners is a mine of knowledge concerning medical affairs in the Army.

[2] See "Walcheren Expedition, Evidence." Hansard, Vol. XV, 1810.

of these duties could not be brought under the criticism of the Board as a whole. The Physician-General, with a salary of 40s. per diem, was responsible for the choice of physicians, for the supervision of medical drugs, and for the examination of candidates for the posts of physician in the Army. The Surgeon-General, with a salary of 40s. per diem, and also an extra £800 per annum as the holder of the sinecure post of surgeon to Chelsea Hospital, appointed the surgeons for the Army and provided surgical drugs and appliances. He occupied a seat on the Court of Examiners at the College of Surgeons for granting a certificate to hospital mates. He consulted with the authorities on medical matters while the troops were on foreign service, and he received the returns of sick and wounded. The Inspector-General was entrusted with the duties of providing Inspectors of hospitals and hospital mates. He had charge of regimental hospitals, and held the position of surgeon to the staff of the Commander-in-Chief. In addition to his salary of 40s. a day, he received an equivalent amount on account of his position of Controller of Army Hospital Accounts. Finally, he was responsible for the provision of drugs for the Guards regiments, and superintended the education of cadets for hospital mates. To complete the description of this edifice of inconsistencies, it remains to be said that the Guards chose their own surgeons, that the medical department of the Ordnance was a separate concern under the control of an Inspector-General, and that the medical comforts were under the control of the Commissary-General. Finally, all the members of the Board were engaged in active private practice.

Such was the state of the Army Medical Board after its duties had been defined in 1798. Had unanimity prevailed, and had machinery existed whereby the Board as a whole could assume authority over its separate departments, it might have been possible to render the system workable. Unfortunately, however, jealousy reigned, quarrels were of frequent occurrence, and its state could only be described as chaotic. But, in spite of all the manifest imperfections of the Board, one great principle was instituted. The medical examination of all candidates was obligatory, although in the case of surgeons it was only the easy pass examination framed by the Corporation of Surgeons for hospital mates.

The Army Medical Board, therefore, proved to be unworkable, and contained in its system the seeds of death which eventually caused its destruction. Some of its faults may be noticed. The Surgeon-General appointed the regimental surgeons, but the class from which they were chosen, the hospital mates, was under the special authority of the Inspector-General. The Inspectors of Hospitals, who were in a position of superior authority to the regimental surgeons, were appointed by the Inspector-General, while the physicians who held a higher rank than the surgeons, were chosen by the Physician-General, and were placed under the Inspectors.

The hospital system in the Army Medical Department was also a cause of much trouble and jealousy. Originally each regiment had a regimental hospital, under the care of the surgeons, but the Board instituted general hospitals, which were largely staffed by physicians, and the regimental hospitals were depleted in order to fill the general hospitals. Owing, it was claimed, to the want of military medical experience of physicians, the patients were not so well treated as in the regimental hospitals. This battle of the hospitals continued for many years, the chief combatants being the Inspector-General, Mr. Knight, with his lieutenants, Dr. Borland, James McGrigor, Robert Jackson, and Young, on behalf of the regimental hospitals, while the Physician-General and the Surgeon-General enlisted the able services of

Dr. E. N. Bancroft on the side of the general hospitals.[1]

The method adopted by Sir Lucas Pepys, the Physician-General, in appointing physicians, also, caused much discontent in the Army Medical Department. When Sir Lucas assumed control, he at once established the rule that he would appoint as physicians only those who were Licentiates of the College. He followed this plan in defiance of the expressly worded order of the Commander-in-Chief, issued in 1798, which said, " for physicians, a medical degree in an English University or a licence from the College of Physicians, although desirable, must not be considered indispensable." Scarcely any medical men already in the Army held the licence, and consequently the superior posts of physician were given to men who had no previous connection with the Army. Staff surgeons and regimental surgeons, however able, were entirely shut out. Sir Lucas when asked, in his examination before the Commissioners of Military Enquiry, why he adopted this method, could only answer that he regarded a knowledge of the principles of medicine as of more importance than special knowledge of Army medical matters. In all, during his occupancy of the post of Physician-General, he had appointed fourteen physicians, not one of whom had ever served in the Army before. In some cases real injustice was done and the efficiency of the service imperilled.[2] The case of Dr. Wright was an example. This physician had practised for seventeen years in the West Indies, and had paid particular attention to diseases incident to that climate. His scientific attainments were of a high order, and when the expedition under Sir Ralph Abercromby was fitting out Sir Ralph

[1] See for this movement "Parliamentary Papers," Vol. XIV, 1810. Vols. 12, 13, 16, 20, 21, 25, and 27 of the War Office Series in the Public Record Office (W.O. 40) also deal with Reform in the Army Medical Department.

[2] See the evidence of Sir Lucas Pepys "Fifth Report of Commissioners for Military Enquiry, 1808."

was anxious to secure his services, but Sir Lucas refused to appoint him unless he held the licentiate of the College. He even went so far as to say that he felt sure the King would refuse to sign his commission without his recommendation. He indicated another gentleman who held the licence, but who had no experience of practical medicine. Sir Ralph was, however, insistent, and Dr. Wright was appointed over the head of the Physician-General.[1]

As the result of all these causes of complaint the Commissioners of Military Enquiry investigated in 1808 the manner in which the Army Medical Board was performing its functions, and their exhaustive report was responsible for the thorough reorganisation of the Army Medical Service and the inauguration of an era of increased efficiency. In this Fifth Report the Commissioners state that, so far as they can ascertain, the condition of the Army Medical Service had never been the subject of enquiry before. They investigated the whole working of the service, they examined on oath all connected with it, and in the end summed up their conclusions in a masterly report which covered eighty pages. They advised a reconstruction of the Board, so that in future it should be a consultative body with a supreme head assisted by a certain number of other individuals. They pointed out the injustice of the manner of selection for various medical posts, and indicated the way in which this selection should be conducted. Finally they took exception to the loose manner in which the members of the Board had supervised the contracts for drugs and appliances, and recommended the employment of some person skilled in accounts to check them.

When the Report was published it brought forth long letters from Keate, the Surgeon-General, in justification of his conduct, in which he indulged in recriminations

[1] See "Letter to Lord Kenyon," Wells, p. 107.

against Knight, Borland, and McGrigor. He imputed to Knight the desire to encroach upon his special department, and want of ability in the management of his own. The quarrel between Knight and Keate was already acute enough, and these letters only served to accentuate the difference still further, with the result that Knight refused to meet the Physician-General and the Surgeon-General.[1] With this state of affairs existing, the Walcheren Expedition took place and emphasised more pointedly than ever the need for reform.

In November, 1809, the Secretary at War appointed a Committee composed of Generals Trigge, De Lancey, Brownrigg, Calvert, and Colonel Gordon to take into consideration the Report of the Commissioners for Military Enquiry and to give effect to their recommendations. The Committee met on November 28th, and succeeding days, and advised the following changes: 1. That the medical department of the Army should be presided over by a single head, to be called the Director-General, with a salary of £2000 a year. 2. That two others, to be called Principal Inspectors, should be associated with the Director-General in the control of the Department, with a salary of £1200 a year each. 3. That in future all promotions must take place among those already in the Army, with due regard to seniority. 4. That the whole time of the Director-General and the Principal Inspectors should be devoted to their duties. District Surgeons were abolished, and the various grades in the service were settled as follows—Inspectors, Deputy Inspectors, Physicians, Staff-Surgeons, Regimental Surgeons, Assistant Surgeons, and Hospital Mates, with respective salaries of 40s., 20s., 15s., 12s., 7s. 6d., and 6s. 6d. per diem. It was the duty of the Director-General to examine hospital mates as to their professional knowledge, but they were to possess the

[1] For this correspondence, see "Parliamentary Papers," Vol. XIV, 1810, Army Medical Service.

certificates of the Court of Examiners at the College of Surgeons for regimental surgeons. Physicians were to be chosen from Staff Surgeons, or were to be Licentiates of the College of Physicians. The Director-General, however, was empowered to hold in addition such examination as he thought proper. Finally, it was decided that no member of the old Board should be eligible for any of the seats on the new Board.[1]

On February 24th, 1810, these changes were carried into effect, and Dr. John Weir was appointed the first Director-General, with Theodore Gordon and Charles Ker as the first Principal Inspectors. The old Board with its impossible methods was swept away, and a new era began in the Army Medical Service. Weir did not hold his position for long, being succeeded in 1815 by Sir James McGrigor, the glory of Army medicine, and from his assumption of office may be dated the real efficiency of the Service.

While the Committee was considering the Report of the Commissioners for Military Enquiry, Sir Lucas Pepys and Thomas Keate wrote several letters to the Secretary at War, in which they complained that they were not consulted with regard to the proposed changes. Sir Lucas especially addressed communications to Lord Palmerston, which must be pronounced to be ill-advised, and in questionable taste. He began by doubting the rumour that he would not be reappointed, and claimed that as he had been appointed by the King it would be an encroachment upon the royal prerogative to supersede him. He spoke in terms of disparagement of Dr. Weir, who was reported to be chosen to fill the position of Director-General, and hinted that, being between sixty and seventy years of age, he was too old for the post. This was strange as coming from a man

[1] The findings of the Committee, together with the correspondence of Keate and Pepys will be found in "Parliamentary Papers," Vol. XIV, 1810, Army Medical Service.

in his sixty-ninth year. Pepys also asserted that, to his knowledge, he had never been remiss in the performance of the duties of his office; but how he reconciled this statement with his refusal to proceed to Walcheren a few months previously it is difficult to say. To all this Palmerston replied in that laconic style so peculiar to him. When Sir Lucas found that it had been definitely decided that he should be superseded—he was not given the option of resigning—he wrote humbly asking that his case might be considered with reference to a pension. This request was granted to him and his former colleagues, and the Army Medical Service embarked upon its new career.

It has often been stated that the Army Medical Board was deposed on account of its shortcomings with regard to the Walcheren Expedition. This is a mistake, for the Commissioners for Military Enquiry had printed their Report before the Expedition was even thought of, and it was on that Report alone that a change was decided upon. The Walcheren Expedition was a coincidence merely which still further confirmed the authorities in their determination to effect a radical change.

But while salutary reform in the direction and control of the Army Medical Department was making headway an important advance had already taken place in the knowledge of medical conditions as they existed in the Army. Sir John Pringle may justly claim to be the father of military medicine, for he gave the first impetus to the study of this subject by the publication, in 1752, of his book, "Diseases in the Army." The incessant wars in which at that time this country became engaged afforded great opportunities for the acquirement of experience in this particular branch of medicine, and of these Pringle availed himself to the fullest extent. The appearance of Pringle's book marks the first attempt to systematise the subject, and to place it on a sure foundation. The work is based on the experience of Pringle while engaged as Physician-General to Forces during the campaigns of 1742–48 in Flanders, Germany, and Scotland. This shrewd observer collected facts concerning the incidence of disease in the Army, the effects of climate and locality, and the influence of variations of temperature and moisture on the health of the troops while engaged on active service.

It is an appalling tale of serious disease constantly following the footsteps of the Army, destroying its efficiency, and producing havoc in its ranks, compared with which losses in battle were trivial. The chief diseases responsible for these losses in effectives were dysenteries, remitting or bilious autumnal fevers, hospital fever, or typhus, besides pneumonias, pleurisies, and rheumatisms, which were of frequent occurrence. Apparently hospital fever or typhus was present in every hospital where soldiers were crowded together, lying on straw which soon became rotten, and constantly breathing the pestilential air, while in the open camp this disease scarcely ever attacked them. For the prevention of these diseases, Pringle advocated the removal of the sick to small regimental hospitals, rather than crowding them together in the large general hospitals. He also laid much stress on the importance of fresh air, dryness, and warmth, and on the necessity for frequently changing the ground on which the camp was pitched.

He studied with great care the climatic conditions, and the endemic diseases of the countries passed through by the troops. In particular he described at length[1] the insalubrity of the island of Walcheren, and, sixty years later, had the Government paid attention to his advice, the disaster of 1809 would have been averted. For many years Pringle's book enjoyed a wide popularity; it was translated into many foreign languages, and several editions were called for, the last being issued in 1810. In

[1] See pp. 6–8, 58, and 171.

fact Pringle was the first to dignify disease in the Army as a special subject, and he may be regarded as the " doyen " of all the long line of eminent men who have worked at this special branch of medical science.

Twelve years after the appearance of Pringle's work, Richard Brocklesby published his " Economical and Medical Observations tending to the Improvement of Military Hospitals,"[1] a book scarcely less important, but far less widely known, than its great forerunner from the pen of Pringle. Brocklesby was a fearless writer, and, as the lifelong friend and admirer of the great Burke, it was only to be expected that his energies would be directed towards the reform of abuses. This was the aim of his book, and it is refreshing to read his spirited attack upon the state of the Army hospitals and the negligence displayed by those responsible for the health of the troops. It required no little courage for a physician to the Army to assail the imperfections of the system and its exponents, but Brocklesby threw caution to the winds and risked his position rather than allow what he conceived to be abuses to pass without comment. He had high ideals as to the duties of doctors and commanders towards those over whom they were placed in control, and he gave his opinions in no uncertain manner.

Apart from the excellent style of the book the observations contained therein are often far in advance of the times. Brocklesby was the first to point out and carry into practice the principle that hospital fever or, as we know it now, typhus, could only be checked by admitting abundant fresh air into the hospitals. At Sandy Heath, near Ripley, and at Winchester, he caused to be constructed temporary hospitals cut out of the chalk and sand in such a way that they admitted a constant current of fresh air, with the result that the

[1] The copy in the College library is of peculiar interest, for it contains corrections for a new edition in the author's handwriting.

fearful epidemic, which had hitherto raged in those places, quickly subsided. His contempt for the plans of existing hospitals at Hilsea and Chatham was undisguised. He also attacked the methods in vogue of commandeering while on active service small cottages to serve as hospitals, which were expected to accommodate forty sick men, although they were constructed originally to house a family of five or six people.

Concerning the organisation of the Army Medical Service he was no less outspoken. He held strongly the view that, since most of the disease in the Army was medical, physicians should have supreme control, and that to them should be given the work of examining candidates for the post of hospital mate. For the surgeons he had no regard, and his strictures concerning their want of education are certainly severe, although he is careful to point out that he is attacking a class and not individuals, some of whom he excepts by name. He was of opinion that the surgeon of a regiment should occupy a position immediately after the field officers, and that both should work together for the preservation of the health of the troops. In the matter of medical knowledge, Brocklesby showed himself to be a most widely read and accomplished physician, and his views upon therapeutics are eminently practical and free from the somewhat nauseous empiricism which tinged the treatment of those days. He was the first to advocate the view that the College of Physicians, through the Censors, should examine those who wished to enter the Army Medical Service, and this probably influenced Pepys in the course he subsequently took.

Other physicians wrote concerning military medicine, notably Donald Monro,[1] but none of them exercised

[1] See "An Account of the Diseases of the British Military Hospitals in Germany," 1764, and "Observations on the Means of Preserving the Health of Soldiers," 1780. An excellent and exhaustive review of works on military medicine in this country, from the earliest times, will be found

such a profound influence upon the subject as Pringle and Brocklesby. The work of these men was, no doubt, responsible for much of the progress made in this field of medicine, but it would have had little effect had it not been for the unremitting endeavours to secure departmental reform that came from within. The names of McGrigor, Borland, Jackson, and Young are closely associated with this movement, and it was largely owing to their ceaseless activities that the Commissioners of Military Enquiry were induced to examine the condition of the Army Medical Service in 1808. Their epoch-making Report resulted in the first steps being taken to place the service on a sound basis, and was the beginning of better days for the Army doctor and the soldier under his care. The advent of Sir James McGrigor as Director-General of the Army Medical Service in 1815 marked the inception of a new era. This able man infused into the service fresh ideas, and during the long period he held office his sole aim was efficiency. He decided that the enormous amount of clinical material should not be wasted, and to this end he compelled all surgeons to make careful reports of epidemics and diseases coming under their notice. All this was collected and arranged in some 350 folio volumes, a worthy monument to his industry and ability. Portions of these manuscripts were eventually published, but much of it is not now available, for it has been destroyed with other documents not thought important enough for preservation.

The above account, then, is a brief outline of the history of the development of the Army Medical Service during the reign of George III. It has been shown that at the beginning of the reign it hardly existed as a

in a "A Concise View of the Progress of Military Medical Literature in this Country," James Irving, M.D., Edinburgh. Stark and Co., 1846. These reviews appeared in the "Edinburgh Medical and Surgical Journal," No. 163.

service, and was under no very efficient control. The great work of Pringle and Brocklesby, who did so much to make military medicine a distinctive branch, has been described, and the causes which were responsible for the Report of the Commissioners for Military Enquiry in 1808 have been traced. After effect had been given to the findings of the Commissioners came Sir James McGrigor, the prince of all Directors-General, and from the time he assumed control may be dated the modern Army Medical Service. Although the Army Medical Service has passed through many vicissitudes since then, the main principles of control initiated by McGrigor have not undergone any fundamental change.

THE WALCHEREN EXPEDITION

In the description just given of the development of the Army Medical Service allusion has been made to the Walcheren Expedition, and since, from a medical point of view, it was a most important military undertaking, it becomes necessary to devote space to its consideration. The disasters which befell this venture were so intimately connected with medical science that it is almost impossible for the historian unacquainted with medicine to write an adequate account of the expedition. In a few short weeks disease swept off, or rendered incapable of military service, a fine army of 40,000 men. Medical reputations were made and blasted, and the evils of divided and incompetent medical control were made abundantly clear. The annals of the British Army contain many instances of the terrible havoc caused by epidemic disease, but it may be doubted if a more appalling tale of disaster produced by sickness and protracted by the supineness of the high medical authorities has ever been recorded. Sickness amongst the troops and inability to cope with it occupied a very considerable part of the despatches of the Commanders-in-Chief, and the tone running through them all was one of failure, hopelessness, and panic.

The medical history of the expedition may be said to have begun with the capture of Flushing on August 15th, 1809, for at about that time sickness in an unusual degree began to be recorded among the troops quartered in South Beveland. The disease rapidly assumed alarming proportions, and by September 10th, when Lord Chatham returned with part of the Army, leaving 16,000 men to hold the island of Walcheren, 8000 of these were on the sick list. The diagnosis of the complaint presented no difficulty; it was clearly miasmatic in origin, and such as might be expected from a residence in the swampy islands of Beveland and Walcheren during the summer and autumn. Indeed, these islands had for a long time borne an evil reputation as being the most fever-ridden places in Europe. There was ample evidence of this, for, sixty years before, Sir John Pringle had given a full description of the complaint as it occurred in these same islands.

Much has been written concerning the conditions existing in Walcheren, but the most complete picture of the state of the Army, and the climate, will be found in a letter written on September 11th by Mr. John Webbe, the Inspector of Hospitals. He says: "Independent of the existing records of the unhealthiness of Zealand, every object around us depicts it in the most forcible manner. The bottom of every canal that has direct communication with the sea is thickly covered with an ooze which, when the tide is out, emits a most offensive effluvia. Every ditch is filled with water which is loaded with animal and vegetable substances in a state of putrefaction, and the whole island is so flat and near the sea that a large proportion of it is little better than a swamp, and there is scarcely a place where water of a tolerably good quality can be procured. The effect of all these causes of disease is strongly marked in the inhabitants, the greater part of whom are pale and listless. The endemic disease of this country, remittent and intermittent fevers, begins to appear about the middle of August and continues to prevail until the frosty weather checks the exhalation from the earth, gives tone to the debilitated frames of the people, and stops thereby the further progress of the complaints. It is computed that nearly a third of the inhabitants is attacked with fever every sickly season. . . . The fever which now unhappily prevails in the Army first appeared among the battalions cantoned in South Beveland, and only began to demonstrate its influence here about the time that Flushing surrendered. The rapidity with which the disease has extended itself during the short period that has elapsed is almost unexampled in the history of any military operations. . . . A considerable number of cases have assumed a more serious form, and have degenerated into that species of low fever which often prevails in jails and other ill-ventilated places in England. As the progress of the mischief is much greater than could rationally have been calculated upon, . . . it must be an inevitable consequence of the British troops remaining in Walcheren that a very considerable loss must be sustained."[1]

Such was the state of the Army in Walcheren on September 11th, and time was to show that Webbe's gloomy forebodings were amply justified. Three days after writing his letter he was stricken down with the fever, and the duty of supreme direction fell upon Francis Burrows, the next in seniority after death had removed Mr. Aveling. The necessity for more doctors became urgent, and on September 14th one staff surgeon and three hospital mates arrived, with the excuse from

[1] For this letter, and the facts upon which this account of the Walcheren Expedition is based, see "Papers Presented to Parliament Concerning the Expedition to Walcheren," 1810, and "The Evidence taken before the House of Commons regarding Walcheren," in Hansard, Vols. XV and XVI.

the Army Medical Board that the war in the peninsula had made such excessive demands upon the supply of surgeons as to render it impossible to send more. The condition of the Army was now deplorable, and the despatches of the Commander, Sir Eyre Coote, dealt with little else than the ever-increasing sickness. Out of an army of sixteen thousand men no less than half were in hospital. The accommodation for the sick was of the worst description, and houses and churches in Flushing, the roofs of which had been destroyed by the bombardment, did duty as hospitals. There were no convalescent hospitals; the supply of blankets, wines, and medicines began to fail, and on September 23rd, Sir Eyre Coote reported that only three hundred pounds of bark remained in store. Typhus fever now made its appearance, and it became evident that strong measures were necessary to cope with this dangerous condition.

The Government at last became alarmed, and in response to the urgent solicitations of Sir Eyre Coote, they requested Sir Lucas Pepys, the Physician-General, and Mr. Keate, the Surgeon-General, to proceed to Walcheren to deal with the terrible sickness which existed in that island. But, to the astonishment of all, Sir Lucas begged to be excused on the ground that he, the Physician-General to the Army, "knew nothing about the investigation of camp and contagious disease"! Keate also refused for the reason that "he conceived he would be of greater use at home." In this dilemma the Government appointed a medical commission, composed of Sir Gilbert Blane, with the title of Acting Physician-General, Dr. James Borland, and Dr. William Lempriere, who were instructed to proceed to Walcheren and report upon the malady prevalent there. In addition they appointed Dr. James McGrigor Inspector-General of Hospitals. Blane and McGrigor arrived on September 30th, and at once made a close examination of the conditions as they existed. They found the roofless churches, houses, and other buildings crowded with sick men, and every day bringing fresh cases in hundreds. They found the medical staff quite insufficient to cope with the work, and the stock of medicines and medical comforts almost exhausted, while, pervading all, they found an atmosphere of paralysis, panic, and despair.

The minds of Blane and McGrigor were soon made up as to the course to be pursued, and on October 1st they addressed a joint letter to Sir Eyre Coote, embodying the measures they judged suitable for the amelioration of this distressing state of affairs. As a first precaution they recommended that about six thousand sick men should be shipped to England in ships of the line, since transports were inadequate. Sir Eyre Coote accepted this suggestion, and during the month of October the evacuation of the hospitals proceeded, with the result that for the first time the depleted medical staff was in a position to cope with the daily influx of sick soldiers.

Blane and his two colleagues returned home on October 10th, but McGrigor remained in supreme charge of all the medical arrangements. Here, he laid the foundation of his immense reputation, and by his energy and sagacity quickly changed the state of medical chaos into one of tolerable efficiency. Sir Eyre Coote gave up the command of the Army on October 29th, and was succeeded by General Don, the third commander to occupy this unenviable position in four months. It was a sorry Army he was called upon to command, for he reported that he had only 4534 men fit for duty, of which about one-third was unfit for considerable exertion. But the agony of Walcheren was soon to be terminated, for the Government decided to evacuate the island. On December 9th the poor remains of the Army embarked; on December 23rd all the heavy ordnance followed, and thus ended the famous expedition.

An exhaustive enquiry took place in 1810, by a Committee of the House of Commons, and the examination of the medical men connected with the expedition revealed an extraordinary state of divided control. The evidence of the members of the Army Medical Board and other doctors showed that the authorities had never consulted the Board with reference to the condition in Walcheren until the sickness began to be excessive. Indeed, until the expedition arrived in the Scheldt, the Board was ignorant of its destination and, therefore, no special provision was made to counteract the dangers of the climate. Although it was proved that the medicines ran dangerously short, there was no evidence to show that the troops were ever in actual want. Blankets and other medical comforts were certainly in insufficient supply, and there was a totally inadequate medical staff to deal with the enormous amount of sickness, although some half-hearted attempts appear to have been made to remedy this defect. In fact the chief blame that could be attached to the Board was that, when the amount of sickness became known, it exhibited a supineness in grappling with the difficulty which nothing could excuse. No measures taken before the expedition started would have had any great effect upon the sickness, for the disease was malaria, which was endemic in Walcheren at the time the Army landed. With the exception of some cases of typhus it was the sole cause responsible for the sickness, and removal from the evil climatic influences was the only remedy.

Many writers when dealing with the medical mission of Sir Gilbert Blane to Walcheren have assigned to him alone the credit, and have claimed for him a position that appears to be not altogether supported by an examination of the facts. They have made it appear that Blane alone was sent out to Walcheren, that he alone made a report to the Government which led to the island being abandoned, and that he alone was thanked for his services. What really happened was as follows: In letters dated September 24th and 26th,[1] the Commander-in-Chief requested Sir Lucas Pepys, with two other physicians of eminence, to proceed to Walcheren "to examine further into the malady prevalent in that island, and to report their opinion thereupon." As has already been stated, Sir Lucas begged to be excused, and Blane was appointed head of the Commission, with the title of Acting Physician-General. The other two members of the Commission were Dr. James Borland and Dr. William Lempriere. Blane reached Walcheren on September 30th, but Borland and Lempriere did not arrive until October 5th. Then a strange thing happened. Blane did not wait for the arrival of his colleagues, nor did he consult with them for some days after, but on October 3rd, 6th, and 9th, he sent letters to Sir Lucas, in which he dealt with the sickness on the island on his own responsibility.[2] Sir Lucas transmitted these letters to the Secretary at War, who regarded this proceeding on the part of Blane as improper, for he ordered Sir Lucas Pepys to be "apprised that Dr. Blane's reports are not to supersede the report that he, in conjunction with Drs. Borland and Lempriere, has been instructed to make concerning the malady prevalent on the island."[3] It is possible that these letters were sent by Blane to Sir Lucas at the latter's suggestion, for after the surprise occasioned by his refusal to proceed to Walcheren, he would naturally desire to be the medium of transmitting first

[1] See "Papers Presented to Parliament Concerning the Expedition to Walcheren," 1810. Letters 67 and 67 E.

[2] See Letters 97, 103, and 110 E, in "Papers Presented to Parliament Concerning Walcheren," 1810.

[3] See Letter 97 E.

hand to the Secretary at War any information regarding the sickness. But while these somewhat subterranean methods were being practised by Blane, the Commission was making its official report. This report was signed on October 10th by the three members of the Commission,[1] and on October 17th the Commander-in-Chief dissolved the Commission, transmitting at the same time the thanks of the Secretary at War for their services.[2] Sir Lucas Pepys evidently sent to Blane the letter of the Secretary at War, in which he refused to allow the letters to supersede the Official Report, for on October 10th Blane wrote to Pepys,[3] and excused himself for going behind the backs of his colleagues on the grounds of their late arrival, and the pressing nature of the business. These excuses appear to be somewhat insufficient, nor was it a graceful act on the part of Blane to call special attention to the assistance he had received from Dr. Lempriere, while omitting altogether the name of Borland. But Borland was not liked by the Army Medical Board, for he was a reformer, and that is perhaps the reason for the omission of his name.

The above is the history of the medical communications made by Blane and the other members of the Commission. In them all there is not a single suggestion that the island should be evacuated. On the contrary, in Section 3 of the Official Report a method is advocated for further garrisoning the island with freedom from sickness. It says: "We presume to recommend to His Majesty's Government, in case the retention of the island should be determined on, to reinforce the garrison very early in the winter." Indeed, from a perusal of the papers relative to the expedition and presented to Parliament in 1810,[4] it is evident that the reason for the abandonment of the

[1] See Letter 104 E. [2] See Letter 109 E. [3] See Letter 110 E.
[4] See Hansard, Vol. XV, 1810.

island was entirely political. This is set out clearly in a despatch from Lord Liverpool to General Don on October 27th, 1809. In that despatch it will be seen that the retention of the island of Walcheren was held to be useless after the peace between Austria and France had been signed on October 14th. While the negotiations begun between Austria and France after the armistice of Zynam dragged on, the occupation of Walcheren was clearly a help to Austria, but already the situation of the British troops was precarious. Bernadotte had arrived in Antwerp with a considerable army, and with Napoleon's forces set free by the signing of the peace it became madness to think of holding the island against such overwhelming strength. It was, therefore, of necessity given up.

It would appear, then, that the account generally given of Blane's position with regard to the Walcheren Expedition is not quite correct. Too much importance has been attached to the part he played, and the names of his colleagues have been, unwittingly, no doubt, suppressed. That his services were most meritorious cannot be denied, and when Sir Lucas Pepys failed to rise to the occasion, it is doubtful if a more competent man could have been found to lead a Commission engaged upon such a vital medical matter.[1]

[1] Blane received £1500 for his visit to Walcheren, but Sir Lucas Pepys was not consulted concerning this grant. The matter was referred to Sir Henry Halford, who suggested the above sum. See "Life of Sir Henry Halford," by Munk, p. 49.

CHAPTER IV

THE NAVAL MEDICAL SERVICE—FAMOUS SICK-BEDS

In order to complete the consideration of Medicine in relation to the State during the reign of George III, the conditions existing in the Naval Medical Service have still to be described.

Materials for the study of the early history of medicine in the Navy are extremely scanty, and it is not possible to describe with any degree of exactness the phases through which it passed until it became an established branch of the Service. Records from comparatively early times do, however, exist which show that physicians and surgeons were appointed from time to time to attend the commanders of various naval expeditions, and presumably to advise them concerning medical questions. One of the first of these appointments, if not actually the first, was that of Roger Marbeck, a Fellow, and the first Registrar of the College of Physicians, who was appointed to attend on the Lord High Admiral Howard in his expedition to Cadiz in 1596. In the British Museum will be found a manuscript of Marbeck, in which he gives an account of his adventures, and this may be regarded as the first report in existence dealing with the medical service of the Navy.[1] In the following year (1597) Henry Atkins, a President of the College of Physicians, was appointed to the expedition of the Earl of Essex to Spain. The agonies of sea-sickness, however, only permitted him to go as far as Plymouth, where he

[1] B.M., Add. MSS. "A briefe and True discourse of the late Honourable Voyage in to Spaine," by Dr. Marbeck.

was landed in an exhausted condition, and his place was taken by Thomas Moundford, another President of the College of Physicians.[1]

In Cromwellian times it became the practice to appoint physicians to naval expeditions proceeding to foreign waters, and the duties attached to these appointments referred more to the care of the sick on board than to the care of the health of the commander of the expedition. Thus, Paul de Laune was appointed by Cromwell as physician to the Fleet proceeding to Jamaica under Penn and Venables. Soon after this the practice became established, and physicians and surgeons were regularly appointed to most of the warships in commission.[2]

Early in the eighteenth century medical affairs in the Navy were under the control of the "Sick and Hurt Board," which was composed of medical and lay members. From an inspection of the minutes of this Board in the Public Record Office it does not appear that the authority conferred upon it was very ample, and for the most part its functions were advisory, but even then, only when applied to by other Naval departments.[3] Indeed, at this time little care was taken of the health of seamen on whom depended the safety of these islands, and such solicitude as existed for their medical welfare was dependent almost entirely upon the energy and conscientiousness of individual naval surgeons. The standard of medical education required was of the lowest kind; they were obliged to provide their own drugs and instruments, and the authorities made no attempt to raise the medical service. But the work of the two great pioneers, James Lind and Gilbert

[1] See "Munk's Roll" for the accounts of Marbeck, Atkins, and Moundford.

[2] See "Munk's Roll" for the account of Paul de Laune.

[3] See "Minutes of the Sick and Hurt Board," Admiralty Series, Public Record Office.

Blane, produced a complete reformation in the Naval Medical Service, and it is not too much to say that the whole of the improvement in Naval Medicine which took place during the reign must be attributed to the work of these great men. On account of the great influence they exercised over medical progress in the Navy it will be necessary to examine their writings.

To Lind perhaps belongs the greater honour, for his was the first definite attempt to improve the position of medicine and hygiene in the Navy. In 1754 he published his work on scurvy, a disease with which he was fully acquainted from the practical point of view. Previous to him, many writers had, it is true, dealt with the subject, but in most of the accounts given no clear and precise description of the clinical features of the complaint can be found. Lind sketched with really masterly hand the special features of this disease, and so ably did he delineate the picture that his description has been followed ever since. But he did more, he indicated for the first time the principles of treatment of scurvy, and showed that, provided the proper anti-scorbutics were carried on board ship, its terrible ravages would very soon become unknown. His wise advice, however, fell upon unheeding ears, and many years were to elapse before scurvy on board ship ceased to limit the naval and mercantile activities of this country.

In 1757 Lind published "An Essay on the most Effectual Means of Preserving the Health of Seamen." The book is not remarkable for its literary style, but is, nevertheless, full of shrewd observations and practical suggestions founded on an extensive acquaintance with disease on board ship. It is one of the most practical books ever written, and it is astonishing how true, even to-day, are many of the observations it contains. His recommendations concerning the care of the health of seamen, his insistence on the necessity for taking bark as a precautionary measure against miasmatic fevers, his remarks regarding hospitals on board ship, and the prevention of infection, had they been attended to, would have saved the lives of thousands of sailors. Probably, however, he was aware of the amount of prejudice his innovations would encounter, and this is the reason why his wise counsels are couched in a somewhat differential tone.

Lind was essentially a pioneer in naval medicine and hygiene. In an age when no thought was given to the care of seamen on board fighting ships, when harsh and repressive discipline was common, he had the courage to point out to the authorities the importance of conserving the health of those on whom the country depended for its defence. His work was epoch making, and from the time that he wrote the attention of the Navy Board was tardily drawn to this important subject. The impetus thus given gained force in succeeding years, until a better state of health in the Service was reached.

If it be true that Lind sowed the seed of medical and hygienic reform in the Navy, it is equally true that Blane tended and garnered the grain, and it is doubtful whether the principles introduced by Lind could have obtained such wide acceptance without his powerful support. Blane was eminently fitted for such work; he was possessed of a most logical mind, a determined yet cautious spirit, and the ardour of a true reformer. He brought these qualities to bear on his work, and when he resigned the chief medical direction of the Navy in 1802 a brighter era of medical progress and efficiency had already dawned.

In 1785 Blane published his book, "Observations on the Diseases of Seamen," and it quickly ran through many editions. The plan of the work bears a somewhat close similarity to that of Lind. Its literary style is easy, almost graceful, and the method, true to the nationality of the author, is mainly deductive. But the chief excellence of the work is its foundation on a wide clinical experience. Blane had little sympathy with mere theory, and in his preface he writes: "The theoretical doctrines of physic have generally no better foundation than hypothesis, and have taken their colour from the prevailing philosophy of the times." The book is divided up into three sections. The first gives a detailed account of the sickness in the Fleet under the command of Lord Rodney while cruising in the West Indies from 1781 to 1783, and to which Fleet Blane was appointed as physician in charge. He ordered the surgeons of ships to take complete notes of the cases, and to furnish exact returns. These results he compiled, and for the first time almost made use of the statistical method in a manner simple yet correct. Although Blane's statistics would by no means satisfy an actuary, still his logical mind kept him clear of those pitfalls in figures and their manipulation into which our profession is so prone to stumble. The net result of his tables was that the annual mortality in the Fleet from disease amounted to 125 per 1000; not an excessive mortality when judged by the standards of those times.

The second section of the book deals with the causes and prevention of disease, and here Blane frankly admits that much of the subject matter is derived from Lind. Indeed, in this section, it is Blane the disciple who is advocating the principles of the master. In the third division of the work observations on fevers are given, and, from the point of view of clinical acumen, this part is the most able and original of all.[1]

The work of Blane and Lind had a profound effect upon the Naval Medical Service, and it stimulated surgeons to devote their attention to the medical needs

[1] For further information concerning the career of Blane see an excellent memoir by Sir Humphry Rolleston, published in the Journal of the Royal Naval Medical Service in 1916.

of those placed under their care. But Blane and Lind were not the only pioneers in this field. The labours of Thomas Trotter,[1] in the direction of a more efficient medical service in the Navy, and towards improvement in the Naval Hospitals, although scarcely less important than those of Blane, were marred by a disposition to attack the ruling powers for their failure to promote reforms. Robert Robertson, a Licentiate of the College of Physicians, was another reformer who did much to quicken the sense of the Navy Board towards the imperfection of the Naval Medical Service.[2]

Not only were surgeons stimulated to fresh activity by the work of these men, but the Naval authorities began to show interest in the subject of the preservation of the health of seamen, and in 1795 a step was taken by the Navy Board which had far-reaching effects. In that year Lord Spencer, the First Lord of the Admiralty, reconstructed the old Sick and Hurt Board, and, under the name of the Commissioners for Sick and Wounded, set up an authority composed of two physicians and one civil member. To these he delegated the direction of all medical matters in the Navy, and for the first time medical men were responsible for the Naval Medical Service. Dr. Robert Blair and Dr. Gilbert Blane were the two medical Commissioners, and Sir William Gibbons was the civil representative. Blair, however, soon retired, and was succeeded by Blane, who at once began to put into practice the principles he had advocated years before. In all, he remained seven years in supreme control of the medical service in the Navy, and when, in 1802, he retired, the Naval Medical Service had been thoroughly regenerated, abuses had been modified or removed,

[1] See "Medicina Nautica," Thomas Trotter, 1797.

[2] See "A Physical Journal kept on board the "Rainbow," 1779. "Observations on Jail, Hospital, or Ship Fever," 1779. "An Essay on Fevers," 1790.

and the way was left clear for progress on prudent lines.

Blane was succeeded by John Harness, who had been appointed a Commissioner in 1800, and he, with organising ability superior even to that of his predecessor, carried forward still further the work of reform. At this time it was felt that the work of the medical department of the Navy was onerous enough to demand the undivided attention of the Commissioners, and it was therefore decreed that they should not engage in private practice. It was soon, however, found that the Commissioners for Sick and Wounded were not sufficiently in touch with the other departments in the Admiralty, and in 1806 the Board was abolished. The functions of the Board were now performed by the Senior Medical Commissioner who sat at the Transport Board, and thus the control of medical matters was vested in one head. Inspectors of Naval Hospitals were appointed in 1804, who acted under the direction of the Medical Commissioner, and in 1817 the Medical Commissioner was again transferred, this time to the Victualling Board, but his functions were the same. Besides Harness, John Weir and Andrew Baird shared in the work, and at the end of the reign of George III, the principles of medical control in the Navy under one authority were well established and have served as the model for all subsequent changes.[1]

The review of medical effort during the reign is now completed, and it is proposed to devote the remaining pages to an account of the scenes taking place around some famous sick-beds when George III was king. It has been urged that a consideration of the illnesses and deaths of eminent personages does nothing to

[1] For most of the facts concerning the development of the Naval Medical Service, use has been made of the evidence of John Harness before the Commissioners of Military Enquiry in 1808, which deals fully with the history of the movement.

advance the knowledge of medicine; that it feeds only a morbid curiosity which good taste often demands should be left unsatisfied. While admitting, however, some show of justice in this criticism, especially when applied to the uninstructed, it may be asserted that the subject of the history of medicine should embrace this special feature, and that a useful purpose will be served by its study. Biographers, however able in a literary sense, have rarely possessed the expert knowledge necessary for a truthful account of the illnesses and deaths of their heroes. On account of this deficiency they have often committed ludicrous errors, and have built up a medical nomenclature and pathology peculiarly their own, of which "brain fever," the beauty, and even pleasure, of death from consumption, and the estimation of a man's large-heartedness from the amount of cardiac hypertrophy found, are some examples.

There are good reasons for an investigation of this kind by those skilled in medicine. In periods of ill-health a man, however great, cannot exercise to the full his mental powers, and it becomes the province of the physician to determine how far bodily and mental ailments have influenced judgment and action. Crises in history and unaccountable lapses of great figures in the world may often be explained by an enquiry into the state of health. Then, the last spoken words of people when "in extremis" have always exercised a fascination over the minds of those who read biography; but the physician knows the amount of value to be attached to such utterances at a time when the higher processes of the brain have often ceased to be in active operation.

After this justification, therefore, it is proposed to describe the illnesses of a few of the more distinguished patients who were attended by physicians in the reign of George III. The first case calling for special consideration is that of the monarch who ruled over England during the whole of the period covered by these lectures.

The family history of George III was by no means good. On his mother's side, who was of the Gotha family, feeble-mindedness, if not actual insanity, had manifested itself. As for his father, Frederic Prince of Wales, all the memoirs and histories of the period in which he lived have failed to disclose one single redeeming feature in his character. He was a degenerate beyond recall. From the first, the intellect of George was essentially dull, and the education provided for him was calculated to accentuate, rather than improve, his mental obtuseness and natural mulish obstinacy. He, therefore, grew up with restricted views and many eccentricities, which a proper education might have softened, although it never could have removed. No king of England was ever on the throne during such mighty intellectual changes. Against every improvement he fought with all his dogged persistence, and although one cherished relic of obsolete feudalism after another was swept away he still failed to profit by the experience.

It has been stated, though on no very sure authority, that George III showed signs of mental derangement as early as 1765. But however that may be, at a levée on October 24th, 1788, it was noticed that the King was strange in his manner and speech. A few days after, undoubted symptoms of insanity appeared which, with varying periods of remission, endured for the remainder of his life. The King's physicians, Dr. Richard Warren, Sir George Baker, Sir Lucas Pepys, and Dr. Revell Reynolds were early in attendance, and on November 26th, at the express command of the Prince of Wales, Dr. Addington was recalled from his retirement to assist his colleagues. He remained in consultation, however, for four days only.

The symptoms of the malady presented no unusual

feature. It was a case of delusional insanity attended with exacerbations of mania followed by periods of melancholia. But insanity in the King raised political considerations of the utmost importance. No precedents existed to guide the two estates of the realm, and until arrangements could be made the whole fabric of government was in abeyance. It was necessary, therefore, to ascertain if the King was really incapable of exercising his regal functions, and further to know how long it would be before recovery took place. Thus it will be seen that the physicians were charged with a serious responsibility, for upon them rested the duty of answering these important questions.

Nor was this all. The state of the two great political parties still further complicated matters and rendered the position of the physicians onerous in the extreme. Both the Whigs and the Tories were agreed that the only way out of the difficulty was to appoint the Prince of Wales as Regent during the incapacity of the King. But the Whigs, headed by Fox, Burke, and Sheridan, regarded the Prince of Wales as their leader, and naturally desired for him a Regency of indefinite duration and ample powers. They were chiefly concerned to make their position secure in the future and not merely for a short period. It was their aim, therefore, to prove out of the mouths of the physicians that it was probable that the King's illness would be of long duration. On the other hand, the Tories, headed by Pitt, knowing that their tenure of power would be ended on the assumption of the regal functions by the Prince of Wales, were equally anxious to limit the Regency both with regard to its powers and duration. They also, like the Whigs, sought to find in the answers of the physicians arguments to support their views. Therefore, however much the physicians might desire to remain aloof from the political turmoil, they were soon to find that they were sucked into the vortex, and were made to take sides often against their inclinations.

In order to ascertain the views of the physicians, they were called and examined before the Privy Council on December 3rd, and the evidence they gave was laid before both Houses of Parliament. Each House then appointed a Committee to examine the physicians at length, and on December 10th and 11th they underwent their examination before these Committees. In the interval two other physicians had been called in; Dr. Francis Willis on the advice of Lord Chancellor Thurlow, and Dr. Thomas Gisborne at the request of the regular physicians in attendance upon the King. The advent of Dr. Willis through the instrumentality of Thurlow savoured somewhat of a political manœuvre, for the Lord Chancellor was a past master in intrigue, and, as will be seen, the answers given by Willis were uniformly on the side of the King's party, of which Thurlow was at that time a pillar. The arrival of Willis on the scene was also viewed with disfavour by the other physicians, for he could scarcely be regarded as a regular practitioner. He was, it is true, a Doctor of Medicine of Oxford, but this had been conferred more to regularise his position as a proprietor of a madhouse than as proof that he had made a serious study of medicine. He was also a Doctor of Divinity, and for a time had been vicar of St. John's, Wapping. For the rest he was a man of most commanding presence, tall and handsome, and had acquired considerable renown on account of his successful treatment of the insane at his madhouse at Gretford, in Lincolnshire. As events were to show, he possessed more experience of lunacy than any of the other physicians, and, throughout, his opinions were more definite, and, therefore, carried greater conviction.[1]

[1] For the few particulars concerning Francis Willis see "The Gentleman's Magazine," 1807, and "Life of George III," Jesse, Vol III. He was educated at Brazenose, graduated M.A., in 1740, and M.D. in 1759. He died in 1807 in his ninetieth year.

The conclusions arrived at as the result of the examination of the physicians may be summarised as follows:—

1. They all agreed that the King was incapable of transacting business.

2. They all expressed hopes of his recovery, especially Addington and Willis, but they would not venture a definite opinion as to when the recovery might be expected. Willis, however, gave the duration as from six weeks to two years.

3. All were questioned as to their experience of mental disease. Pepys and Gisborne confessed to having had little experience. Addington and Willis owned to considerable experience, while Warren, Baker, and Reynolds appealed to such cases as had arisen in their extensive practices spread over many years.

4. None of the physicians could see any signs of convalescence, and none would assign a cause for the attack, except Willis, who thought that too much business, severe exercise, too little sleep, and much abstemiousness were chiefly responsible.[1]

Although these conclusions exhibited much caution on the part of the physicians, evidence was not wanting that already the King's party was looking to Willis as their chief medical support, while the Whigs had fixed upon Dr. Warren as the physician most likely to further their aims. No improvement took place in the King's health, and on January 6th, 1789, Burke pressed for a Committee to enquire concerning it. He stated that, contrary to expectation, the King's health had not improved, and he read Dr. Warren's evidence, given in December, to support his argument that it was possible that the King might not recover. Whether willingly or not, Warren and Willis were now definitely in opposite camps in this bitter contest, and the debate turned

[1] For the evidence of the physicians regarding the King's condition see "Parliamentary History," Vol. XXVII.

upon their medical position and experience. At the mention of Warren's name the party of Pitt made derisive and unseemly noises, and Pitt at once stated that he preferred to rely upon the opinion of Willis, who had more experience of the disease than any of the other physicians, while Warren had scarcely any. Burke and Fox, who were friends of Warren, in reply passed eloquent and stately eulogiums upon his skill and character, and with regard to Dr. Willis, who was so learned in insanity, they asked why Dr. Monro, the superintendent of Bethlem, had not been called in, or as Burke said, "Why not put one doctor of a madhouse against another?" In the end Pitt acceded to this request for the appointment of a Committee of twenty-one members, which took 400 folio pages of evidence.[1]

On January 13th the House considered this report, and again the storm of party conflict revolved around the question of the skill of Warren and Willis. Burke, in heated but majestic language, complained that Warren and Willis had been examined as if they were equal in point of skill. He ended by saying that he did not believe that the King's life was safe in the hands of Willis, who had actually trusted a razor in the King's hand. Sheridan also said that the answers of Dr. Willis were most evasive and prevaricating. Of course the design of this arraignment was to show that the opinion of Willis, who regarded the illness of the King as temporary only, was of little weight. Pitt, on the other hand, with equal vehemence, combated this view, and maintained that the evidence showed that, although the King was incapable of business, the incapacity was only temporary, and that, therefore, an interval merely had to be provided for. With consummate ability, Pitt seized upon the point that three of the physicians were

[1] For the evidence given before this Committee see "House of Commons Journal," 1789.

conversant with the disease, but that Dr. Warren and Sir George Baker were not. He pointed out that the two latter only saw the King for two hours each day, while the others saw him from 3 p.m. to 11 a.m., and Willis more than them all. He held, therefore, that the opinion of those who saw the King most frequently was to be accepted, and those who were with him most of all believed in his recovery. In fact, Pitt supported the view of Willis and placed in him implicit trust. Having thus thrown down the gauntlet, he then dealt the Whigs a parting blow by hinting that Warren was influenced in his opinion by a "high authority," meaning, of course, the Prince of Wales.

Such was the tone of the debates so far as the physicians were concerned. In the end, the Regency Bill was framed in accordance with Pitt's wishes, but it was never put into operation, for, in March, the physicians were able to declare the King recovered from his illness.

The question must now be asked—How far were Warren and Willis actuated by party motives in the opinions they gave? After reading the evidence given, and after considering the political atmosphere which surrounded the sick couch of George III, it appears to be almost impossible to escape from the conclusion that the opinions expressed by the two chief medical opponents were influenced by party spirit. The private associations of the two men also lend some support to that view. Willis, as has been mentioned, was suddenly introduced by Lord Thurlow, and this in itself was suspicious. It has also been stated that Willis was a strong adherent of Pitt in Lincolnshire. Warren was admittedly a personal friend of Burke and Fox, a member of the literary circle which drew its inspiration from Johnson's famous club, and eventually a member of the club itself. It is peculiar, also, that Warren never called in a mental specialist, although in evidence he admitted that he always called in one in cases of this kind. It is true that he did consult Dr. Monro, but he never called him in. Did he fear that Monro would side with the other expert, Willis? No doubt the position of the physicians was most difficult, and perhaps circumstances were too strong for them, but after making all allowance for the delicate nature of their task, the opinions given by Warren and Willis can hardly be exempted from the suspicion of having been tinged with political bias.

But while the House of Commons was contending for the royal power temporarily relinquished by George III, another contest equally bitter was being waged within the royal sick-chamber. Even here the baneful influence of party strife made itself felt, and the position was rendered more difficult by the unworthy squabbles which broke out among the physicians. The regular medical attendants of the King had no experience in the management of a lunatic, and they hesitated to submit their august patient to the ordinary methods of control. The King acted as he pleased, and one night when he became violent, Sir George Baker could not be prevailed upon to suggest to the King that he should retire for the night. Sir George did not reap any advantage from his forbearance, for the King suddenly seized him by the throat and pinned him to the wall. With the advent of Willis, however, matters improved. He understood the management of the insane, as practised in those days, and he applied to the King the usual methods of repression and coercion. Very soon he acquired an ascendency over the monarch, and although he incurred the intense and lasting aversion of his royal patient, he was feared and obeyed. By degrees, the regular physicians were thrust more and more into the background, and Dr. Willis, assisted by his son, Dr. John Willis, assumed complete control of the invalid. The King was soon removed from Windsor to Kew and arrangements were made for his care and treatment. Willis did not hesitate to cause the patient to be confined in a straight waistcoat when he became violent, and it is probable that the King received harsh treatment at the hands of Ernst, the Prussian page of the back-stairs, who acted as chief attendant. The stories, however, of the brutal treatment meted out to George III, during his insanity, are much exaggerated, and gained credence at the time chiefly through the statements made by Lady Harcourt. Her evidence, however, when closely inspected, is full of inaccuracies and is not worthy of implicit trust. All those about the King's person were genuinely sorry for his unhappy position, with one notable exception, his eldest son, the Prince of Wales, and he, the First Gentleman of Europe, had the execrable taste to indulge his undoubted powers of mimicry at the club, in portraying to his satellites the antics and ravings of his afflicted father.

The supercession of the regular physicians by Dr. Willis accentuated the bad feeling which already existed, and bitter quarrels took place over the treatment, and the particular form in which the daily bulletins should be issued. Willis was, of course, anxious to show that the King was progressing towards recovery, while Warren and the others were concerned to paint his condition in more gloomy colours. To make matters worse it was found that Willis was writing on his own authority to Pitt, without consulting the others. On one occasion Willis stated to Pitt that the King was making great progress when, according to the other physicians, the patient had passed a very restless and violent night. Dr. Warren rightly characterised these proceedings as political rather than medical. Court ladies were apparently the medium for communications between the Prince of Wales and the physicians, and on more than one occasion the Prince interfered to have the bulletins altered. But the culminating point was reached one morning when the physicians, on going to see their patient, were confronted with a notice pinned up in the anteroom stating that no one might see the King without the permission of the Doctors Willis! Willis was in supreme authority and he arranged matters as he pleased. But the medical tragedy was drawing to a close; in February the King showed undoubted signs of regaining his reason, and in the following month the physicians were able to declare him capable of transacting business again.

It cannot be said that much credit is due to the regular physicians in attendance for the way in which they managed the King's illness. A perusal of the evidence given leaves the impression that the illness itself and its treatment were matters of secondary importance when compared with the all-absorbing question of the political results to be expected from the illness. Willingly or unwillingly, the physicians, especially Warren and Willis, by the opinions they expressed, served the ends of violently opposed political factions, while the others apparently by their silence acquiesced in the course of conduct adopted. The regular physicians admitted that they knew little or nothing about the treatment of mental disease. Yet, when Willis had been introduced, they failed to take the obvious course of calling in another alienist of approved reputation for their own protection. Both Simmons and Monro were available, but were never summoned, with the result that the King's physicians were relegated to a secondary position at the command of a man they regarded as little better than a quack. It has been the fashion to express contempt for the medical ability of Willis, but it must not be forgotten that he alone had a definite plan for the treatment of the King, that after his arrival haphazard methods gave place to orderly treatment, and that he, of all the physicians, was most confident in his belief that the King would soon recover, a belief that was borne out by future events.

In 1801 the King became again affected, and although the attack was not severe it lasted for about five months. In this attack the Willis family again assumed almost absolute control, and the King was constantly under the supervision of either Dr. John Willis or the reverend Dr. Thomas Willis, who represented their father, Dr. Francis Willis, now prevented by age from being in active attendance. In 1804 a third relapse took place. The more acute symptoms lasted from February to March, but convalescence was not established until some months later. Previous to this attack the King had stated his strong objection to be under the care of the Willis family in case he should have another relapse, and it was, therefore, arranged that he should be attended by Dr. Samuel Foart Simmons, the able physician to St. Luke's Hospital. Dr. Simmons proved to be an excellent choice, and it is probable that for the first time the King had the benefit of really capable and judicious treatment. On both of these occasions he was incapacitated from undertaking public business, but the government of the country was carried on and little was allowed to transpire concerning the illness.

In the three attacks of insanity sustained by George III, an exciting cause can be found in the political crises which immediately preceded them. Before the first attack the King had passed through the disasters which resulted in the separation of the American Colonies, and to this blow was added the effect upon his mind produced by the disgraceful conduct of the heir-apparent with regard to his marriage with Mrs. Fitzherbert. Pitt's determination, in spite of the obstinate opposition of the King, to bring in a bill for the emancipation of the Catholics, and his subsequent resignation, were certainly largely responsible for the King's second attack in 1801, and the trouble arising out of Addington's unstable administration no doubt induced the attack in 1804.

On October 25th, 1810, the King for the fourth time showed acute symptoms of insanity. Indeed, ever since his last attack he had never really recovered, but had been more or less peculiar in his manner. The present attack was severe, and was brought on by the shock the King had sustained by the death of his favourite daughter, the Princess Amelia. The physicians attending the King on this occasion were Dr. Reynolds, Dr. Baillie, Dr. Heberden the younger, Sir Henry Halford, and Dr. Robert Willis. As in the first attack, they were examined before the Privy Council on November 28th and 29th, and before the two Houses on December 14th and 17th. The evidence was interesting, for all the physicians were convinced that the King, although he had had three previous attacks and was in his seventy-second year, would recover, and probably soon. They were pressed to say what experience they had of a man at that period of life recovering, and could give none. Baillie and Heberden bluntly told the Committee that they had no experience of mental disease, while Halford and Reynolds relied on the cases they had seen in private practice. The only expert was Willis, who had succeeded his father, and it was strange that no other specialist was called in. Politics played no part in this examination, for all parties were agreed that a Regency was the only possible way out of the difficulty. The examination cost Reynolds his life, for he was unequal at his time of life to the exertion of standing for hours while giving his evidence. He never recovered from the fatigue and died very soon after. Contrary to the expectations of the physicians, the King never regained his reason, and, after passing ten years in this sad state, died in 1820.

While George III, aged, helpless, and insane, was dying in seclusion in England, in a far-off sea-girt isle death was about to claim the most remarkable example of brain energy that the world has ever produced. For in St. Helena, the great Napoleon, a prisoner, and stripped of all earthly power, was on the point of making his exit. As in the case of George III, his illness is an example of the evil of allowing politics to be blended with the practice of medicine. Indeed, it is not too much to say that Napoleon's complaint was misjudged throughout, almost entirely on account of political influences which obscured the judgments of the medical attendants. It was not the British Authorities only who were responsible for the introduction of politics, for Napoleon himself was equally to blame. The chief question at issue between the French at Longwood and the British Authorities was not the precise nature of the malady of the Emperor, but rather how far climatic influences were responsible for its onset. Whether or not Napoleon suffered from attacks of hepatitis induced by the climate is a debatable subject, but as to the cause of his death there can be no dispute. He died of cancer of the pylorus, which remained undiagnosed until the post-mortem examination was made, although disease of the stomach was surmised a few days before he died. Situated as he was, Napoleon had not at his command medical assistance of a very high order, for the surgeons who attended him were of mediocre talents, and excessively fearful of compromising their position by the expression of medical opinions contrary to the official views.

The lot of kings when stretched upon a bed of sickness is far less enviable than that of humbler mortals. Politics and the august presence of royalty seem to conspire together to paralyse the efforts of physicians, and it may be doubted if the prognosis in cases of illness among kings can ever be regarded in so favourable a light as in those of more lowly beings. The same remarks do not, however, apply to great figures in literature. Indeed, they appear to be able to command all the ability and sympathy of the physicians who attend them. The case of Samuel Johnson illustrates this point, and probably no man was ever treated during his illnesses with such tenderness and ungrudging solicitude by physicians of eminence, who often held opinions widely at variance with those of their patient.

All his life Johnson possessed a warm personal regard for doctors. Many of his friends belonged to that profession, and he had written the lives of Boerhaave, Garth, and Akenside. Several physicians had even enjoyed the honour of being elected members of the literary clubs over which Johnson exercised sway To the club in Ivy Lane Drs. McGhie, Barker, and Bathurst belonged, while at the more celebrated one at "The Turk's Head" in Gerrard Street, two physicians, Dr. George Fordyce and Dr. Nugent were among the members. Besides these, several physicians were close friends of Johnson, and foremost among them were Dr. Thomas Lawrence, Dr. Richard Brocklesby, and Dr. Robert James. For Lawrence, who was a distinguished President of the College, Johnson had a warm affection, and it was in Lawrence's consulting-room that one of the most extraordinary consultations took place. Mrs. Piozzi relates the incident, which occurred in 1781 when Johnson, who was suffering from asthma and dropsy, sought the advice of his friend. It so happened that Lawrence had recently been attacked with hemiplegia and aphasia, and both patient and physician were extremely hard of hearing. In these circumstances any idea of a consultation was out of the question, so, seeing the humour of the situation, they occupied their time by writing punning sentences in Latin to each other.

There was another reason also for the delight Johnson took in the society of doctors. He was a keen amateur student of medicine, and took the greatest interest in his own ailments. His robust temperament made him a strong believer in drastic remedies as opposed to palliatives. The physician could never give Johnson too violent a remedy, and if he faltered the patient made him aware of it by some taunt. In this way he showed his displeasure at the cautious treatment of the great Heberden by referring to him as "timidorum timidissimus." Another habit of Johnson when ill was to supplement the efforts of the physicians by strong measures of his own, and, as we shall see, this ill-judged interference in the end cost him his life.

For many years the health of Johnson was robust, and, with the exception of fits of depression, it could not be said that he suffered from ill-health. As years advanced, however, he began to be troubled with symptoms of bronchitis and emphysema. Breathlessness on exertion became particularly troublesome, and his nights were disturbed by cough, inability to assume a recumbent position, and severe attacks resembling asthma. By the time he had passed the age of sixty other symptoms pointing to grave interference with the circulation, such as palpitation, giddiness, and swelling of the legs, began to make their appearance. For the bronchitis the usual remedies were prescribed, and particularly squills in large doses, but Johnson seemed to obtain more relief from ample and repeated venesections. Opium in large doses was effectual in cutting short the attacks of asthma, but he soon became aware of the danger of continuing its use, and after having taken as much as four grains in a single dose he had the courage to abandon the practice.

Johnson continued to be troubled with these symptoms until June 16th, 1783, when a serious event took place. On that night he went to bed as usual, but in a short time was aroused with, as he described it, "confusion in the head," and was alarmed to find that he had lost the power of speech. His mental faculties, however, were not much impaired, for he could put a prayer into Latin, and could think and reason without difficulty. Although he had not completely lost power of the movements of the right hand, he experienced great difficulty in forming the letters when he tried to write a letter. This letter, which was a request to his friend Dr. Taylor to obtain the assistance of Drs. Heberden and Brocklesby, is in existence, and shows, only too plainly, that, in spite of Johnson's assertion, his mental faculties were impaired by the attack. It contains several repetitions of words, and exhibits curtailment of the power to express thoughts.

While he was waiting for the arrival of the doctors he, as usual, decided to treat himself, and, as he said, " to rouse the vocal organs " he took two glasses of wine. Heberden and Brocklesby now arrived, and at once noticed that Johnson's face was drawn to one side. He had so far recovered that he could speak, though indistinctly, and could repeat fairly well the Lord's Prayer. The doctors learning that the attack was passing off, gave a good prognosis, and their opinion was justified, for on the second day the paralysis had disappeared, and by the fourth day he had entirely recovered the use of speech.

But although Johnson recovered from this attack, it was, in fact, the beginning of diseased conditions which were soon to terminate his life. Towards the end of 1783 dropsy supervened, and the legs and thighs swelled up to an enormous extent. He became seriously alarmed at his state, and set apart a day for fasting and humiliation. To his joy he had the satisfaction of seeing the water in his legs disappear as if by magic. In fact, in twenty-four hours he voided over twenty pints of urine. It must, however, be mentioned that besides the day of fasting and humiliation, Johnson had been taking quantities of diuretics, and perhaps some would argue that these drugs had as much to do with the happy result as the treatment by way of penance. In any case, the dropsy which had persisted for 120 days was gone, and now, with the exception of a slight cough, he enjoyed a measure of health for a limited period.

About this time he did a most unwise thing. Although he had at his command the skill of the ablest medical men that London could produce, and among them were such great names as Heberden, Baker, Pepys, Warren, and Brocklesby, he was persuaded by Boswell to consult by letter the great medical authorities in Edinburgh. He, therefore, detailed the symptoms of his case to Cullen, Alexander Dick, Gillespie, and Monro. The result was what might have been expected. They indicated a line of treatment which interfered with that adopted by the London physicians, and Johnson's time was largely employed in taking incredible quantities of drugs.

In 1784 the dropsy returned, and the stomach began to show signs of derangement. Liberal doses of squills and other diuretics produced some remission, and he was in no great distress until November 8th, 1784, when the dropsy became again formidable. From July 6th to November 8th of this year Johnson recorded his symptoms in a journal, and it is a faithful, if melancholy, account of his last days. But he was now on his death-bed, and the end was to take place very soon. The dropsy had assumed such enormous proportions that Mr. Cruikshank, at the earnest solicitation of Johnson, was requested by the physicians to make incisions in the legs and scrotum to let out the water. This operation was performed on December 11th, and on the morning of the 13th Johnson ordered his servant to hand him a lancet, and with his own hand he made the cuts deeper. In this operation about ten ounces of blood were lost, but it was more than the enfeebled constitution of Johnson could bear. He soon began to sink, and before the day was out he was no more.

Few men, whatever their position in the world, have been attended with such unselfish devotion and consideration. For the physicians who cared for Johnson it was a labour of love, and their attitude on this occasion constitutes one of the bright pages in the history of our profession. Macaulay has stated that the ablest physicians placed their skill at Johnson's disposal and refused to accept fees. That is true, but although moribund, Johnson insisted that a copy of "The Lives of the Poets" should be placed in the coach of each of the distinguished physicians as he left the house.

In connection with the illness and death of Johnson, the library of the College of Physicians possesses a document of the greatest interest in the form of the original report of the post-mortem examination, in the handwriting of the operator, Mr. James Wilson. This document has, it is true, been published in 1849 in the "London Journal of Medicine," but since it is little known, and not very accessible, it may be transcribed. It is as follows :—

"Wednesday, December 15th, 1784, opened the body of Dr. Samuel Johnson for Mr. Cruikshank, in the presence of Drs. Heberden, Brocklesby, Butler, Mr. C., and Mr. White. He died on Monday preceding. About a week before his death Mr. C. by desire of his physicians sacrificed his legs and scrotum, to let out the water which was collected in the cellular membrane of those parts, Dr. Johnson being very impatient to have the waters entirely gone. On the morning of the day he repeated the operation himself and, cutting very deep, lost about ten ounces of blood; he used a lancet for this purpose; he was in too weak a state to survive such an apparently trifling loss. For several years past he had been troubled with asthma, for which he commonly used to take opium, and found that nothing else was of any service to him; he had discontinued, however, this practice some years before he died.

"On opening the cavity of the chest, the lungs did not collapse as they usually do when air is admitted, but remained distended, as if they had lost the power of contraction; the air-cells on the surface of the lungs were also very much enlarged; the right lobe adhered very strongly to the diaphragm; the internal surface of the trachea was somewhat inflamed; no water was found in the cavity of the thorax. The heart was exceedingly large and strong, the valves of the aorta were beginning to ossify; no more fluid than was common was contained in the pericardium. In the abdomen seemed to be incipient peritoneal inflammation and ascites; the liver and spleen were firm and hard; the spleen had almost the feel of cartlidge. A gall stone about the size of a pigeon's head was taken out of the gall bladder; the omentum was exceedingly fat; nothing remarkable was found in the stomach; the folds of the jejunum adhered in several places to one another; there was also a strong adhesion by a long slip between the colon and bladder; the pancreas was remarkably enlarged; the kidney of the left side tolerably good, some hydatids beginning to form on its surface; that of the right side was almost entirely destroyed, and two large hydatids formed in its place. Dr. Johnson never complained of any pain in this part; the left testicle was perfectly sound in structure, but had also a number of hydatids on its surface, containing a fatty gelatinous fluid, the right testicle had hydatids likewise, but the spermatic vein belonging to it was exceedingly enlarged and varicose. The cranium was not opened.

"N.B.—Mr. White, assisting me to sew up the body, pricked his finger with the needle; the next morning he had red lines running up the arm, and a slight attack of fever."

The illnesses responsible for the deaths of eminent Georgians may often be traced to habits, particularly common to that age, of inordinate eating and drinking. A prominent case of this kind is that of Charles James Fox, who was in reality a victim of his own generous and warm-hearted disposition. His upbringing is well known; how at an early age he was encouraged to drink, gamble, and indulge in every kind of wild debauchery by that detestable father, Henry Fox, the first Lord Holland. The wonder is that so much of the noble and chivalrous nature of Charles Fox was preserved after such a terrible tutelage. His constitution must have been splendid. Up to within two years of his death he was a complete stranger to serious illness, and used to boast that a dose of sulphur was sufficient to remove all the ills he had ever known. Most of his nights were spent in gambling at the club, where he consumed oceans of wine, or in the House of Commons, where his vigour and powers of declamation were equalled only by those of Pitt. Until the fifty-fourth year of his age no impairment of health was noticeable, but already the pace had begun to tell, and Fox was about to pay the debt to outraged nature.

In 1804, while at Cheltenham, he complained of a feeling of discomfort over the liver, and was advised to consult a doctor. A peculiarity of his, however, was a strong dislike to speak of his ailments, and still more to allow a medical man to examine him. About a year after this, Lord Lauderdale called his attention to the fact that his abdomen and legs were very swollen. Fox then confided to his friend that for some time past his appetite had failed, that his strength was feeble, and that he was troubled with sickness in the morning. David Pitcairn, Halford, and Moseley were consulted and pronounced the disease to be dropsy. This was self-evident, and was, of course, due to cirrhosis of the liver induced by intemperate living. The accumulation of water in the peritoneal cavity became so considerable that it was deemed necessary to have recourse to tapping, and on Fox's removal to Chiswick a second operation became imperative. On September 7th, 1806, he became much worse, and soon relapsed into a moribund condition. In this state he remained until the 13th, when he expired. At the post-mortem examination it was found that the liver was in an advanced state of cirrhosis, the natural consequence of the irregular life he had led.

In fact, the end of brilliant Charles Fox was similar to that of the common gin-drinker in the back slums. While we deplore the irregularities of his life, we still have in grateful remembrance his manful fight against political oppression, and our sympathies are still moved by the memory of his life-long championship of civil and religious liberty. Perhaps Fox would not be so near to our hearts to-day had he been a paragon of spotless virtue.

The end of Fox's great Parliamentary rival, the austere and immaculate Pitt, took place in the same year, but much obscurity surrounds his illness. There can be no doubt that over-indulgence in alcoholic liquor was in part responsible for Pitt's condition, for all his life he was immoderately fond of port wine. Since Addington recommended liberal quantities of this wine to counteract the weakly constitution of Pitt when a child, responsibility for the habit thus encouraged must rest in part upon that physician's shoulders. Then gout, which laid a heavy hand on all the male members of Pitt's family, did not spare him. To these adverse conditions must also be added the terrible mental strain produced by the unsuccessful struggle in which the country was engaged with Napoleon, and when Austerlitz appeared to be the grave of European liberty, the enfeebled constitution of Pitt sank under the blow, and death became imminent. At about that time he began to waste rapidly, and the stomach rejected the lightest form of nourishment. After a protracted journey from Bath to Putney which caused his physician, Sir Walter Farquhar, much anxiety, Dr. Baillie was called in, and the gravity of the case was clearly recognised. Remedies were of no avail, and in a few days the patient died. It is impossible now to assign the actual cause of death, but the opinion may be hazarded that Pitt suffered from malignant disease, or chronic ulcer, of the stomach.

The cases narrated above are examples of the famous patients attended by physicians in the reign of George III. Space does not permit of the list being extended, but perhaps the instances given will serve to stimulate interest in this special branch of the history of medicine. It must be remembered that the arrangements in the sick-room in those days were not such as we are accustomed to expect at the present time. Skilled nursing was unknown, the sanitary conveniences were neglected, and fresh air was regarded as harmful. Frequently the patient was allowed to rest on a couch, until increasing weakness compelled him to take to his bed, and a considerable latitude was permitted with reference to the kind of nourishment taken.

In concluding this review of the state of medicine during the reign of George III, some considerations may be advanced concerning the advantages of a study of the history of medicine.

In recent years the study of this subject has made great progress, and at most centres, both here and on the Continent, its investigation has become almost a recognised branch of medicine.

Although the days have long since passed when the mere mention of medical history raised a smile of genial sarcasm, many of us would be glad to see a still wider interest shown in the subject. Sound arguments may be advanced in support of this desire. At the present day, the immense range covered by the word "medicine" leaves but little time for the cultivation of extraneous studies which both elevate the mind and increase its usefulness in human life and endeavour. For this reason the title of "physician" is not now so synonymous with culture as it was in former years. Indeed, with the multifarious duties which fall to the lot of physicians in these days, it is wellnigh impossible to expect of them a wide and profound acquaintance with subjects outside the sphere of their immediate and pressing work. But a study of the history of medicine would permit the physician, while still tethered to his life work, to roam in a wide circle into the realms of history, biography, philosophy, and all the activities of the human mind. It would, at least, be a hobby, and so long as a hobby does not overwhelm the main purpose in life, it implies no disgrace, but rather operates as an agent of high recuperative value.

It has been urged that a study of this subject cannot advance our knowledge of present-day medicine. That may be true. But how can knowledge of any part of medicine be complete without an investigation of the early steps taken from hypothesis to accepted fact. The Church, the law, politics, art, and science all have their histories. Why should medicine, the meeting-point of all human emotions, lag behind?

If medical history be deemed worthy to form part of the education of physicians, surely no more fitting place can be found for its abode than the College of Physicians, the ancestral home of physicians for four centuries. The College has founded the FitzPatrick Lectures for the purpose of encouraging the study of the history of medicine, and is thus the first medical body in this country to accord recognition to this particular subject. The connection between the College and medical history is of the most intimate nature, and it is impossible for those belonging to it to remain uninfluenced by its great traditions. There everything around reminds them of the history of British medicine. On the staircase, in the reading-room, and in the Censors' room they gaze on the portraits of physicians who have laboured to advance the knowledge of medicine. The choice and magnificent library contains rich stores contributed by the great master-builders of the past. At the College meetings the Fellows occupy seats once filled by their great predecessors, Heberden, Baillie, Arbuthnot, Friend, Young, and Bright. The Presidential Chair recalls to them the long line of disdinguished physicians who have adorned that eminent position, down to the present occupant who has done so much to encourage learning and the study of the history of medicine. It is a great heritage, and in proof of its vitality, it need only be stated that, while dynasties and empires have risen and crumbled in decay, the Royal College of Physicians is still, after four centuries, at the full tide of its strength and influence.

We cannot afford to neglect the study of this branch of medicine. Veneration for those who have laboured to perfect the knowledge of our art, and the desire to be exactly informed concerning their work make it incumbent upon us to include this subject among those required for a complete medical education.

APPENDIX

THE STATISTICS OF THE MEDICAL PROFESSION 1760–1820

A DETAILED STATEMENT OF THE NUMERICAL STRENGTH OF THE PROFESSION IN 1782

Physicians Resident in London . .	149	
Surgeons	274	
Apothecaries	351	
	——	774
Practitioners Resident in the Provinces .	3560	
Practitioners Resident in Wales . .	125	
	——	3685
Total in England and Wales . .		4459

(Reference, "Medical Register," 1783.)

THE NUMERICAL STRENGTH OF THE PROFESSION

Area	Year	Population	Prac- titioners	Propor- tion
England & Wales	1782	7,814,827	4459	1 in 1752
London	—	650,845	774	1 in 840
England & Wales	1911	36,070,492	25,472	1 in 1416
London	—	4,521,685	6,415	1 in 705

In 1817 it was estimated that 1098 medical practitioners were resident in London, which then had a population of 1,100,000, which gives a proportion of about one medical man to 1000 people.

Since no correct census of the people was taken before 1801 the numbers given before that date are estimates only.

(References, "Medical Register," 1783.
The Census Returns.
"A Picture of the College," 1817.
"Porter's Progress of the Nation.")

THE COMPOSITION OF THE COLLEGE OF PHYSICIANS

1746

Fellows	54	Licentiates	24
In the West End	7	In the West End	7
In the City	34	In the City	13
Elsewhere	13	Elsewhere	4

(An Address to the College, 1747.)

1753

Fellows	41	Licentiates	42

(See "A Letter from a Physician," 1753.)

1782

Fellows	43	Licentiates	74
In the West End	18	In the West End	24
In the City	8	In the City	27
Elsewhere	17	Elsewhere	23

(See "Medical Register," 1783.)

1817

Fellows	89	Licentiates	224
In the West End	38	In the West End	67
In the City	7	In the City	25
Elsewhere	44	Elsewhere	132

(See "A Picture of the College," 1817.)

THE CREATION OF FELLOWS AND LICENTIATES

Year	Fellows admitted	Licentiates admitted
1760–9	17	56
1770–9	13	30
1780–9	17	79
1790–9	21	54
1800–9	25	98
1810–19	35	99
Total for 60 years . .	128	416
Annual Average . .	2.1	6.9

FACILITIES IN LONDON FOR MEDICAL INSTRUCTION, 1783

Lectures on the Theory and Practice of Physic, and Materia Medica.

Dr. Fordyce, at his house in Essex Street, Strand.

Dr. Saunders, at Guy's Hospital.

Dr. Maddocks, at the London Hospital.

Clinical Lectures.

Dr. Fordyce, on cases of patients at St. Thomas's Hospital.

Drs. Saunders and Keir, on cases in Guy's and St. Thomas's.

Dr. Maddocks, on cases in the London Hospital.

Dr. Simmons, on cases at the Westminster General Dispensary.

Lectures on Diseases of Children.

Dr. Andrew Wilson, at his house in Beaufort Buildings.

On Animation.

Dr. Hawes, at his house in Great Eastcheap.

Chemistry Lectures.

Dr. Fordyce, at his House in Essex Street.

Drs. Saunders and Keir, at Guy's Hospital.

Dr. Maddocks, at the London Hospital.

Dr. Bryan Higgins, at his house in Greek Street, Soho.

Philosophy of Chemistry and Natural History.

Dr. Henry Moyes, at Mr. Walker's in George Street, and at the Plasterer's Hall, Aldermanbury.

Lectures on Anatomy and Dissections.

Mr. Cruickshank, at Great Windmill Street.

Dr. R. Maclaurin, at his house in Mark Lane.

Mr. Blizzard, at the London Hospital.

Mr. John Sheldon, at his house in Great Queen Street.

Mr. H. Cline, at St. Thomas's Hospital.

Lectures in Midwifery.

Drs. David Orme and Lowder, at Dr. Lowder's, St. Saviour's Churchyard.

Dr. John Leake, at his house in Craven Street.

Drs. William Osborne and Thomas Denman, in Leicester Street.

Dr. Robert Bland, at his house in St. Alban's Street.

Lectures in Surgery.

Mr. Percival Pott, at St. Bartholomew's Hospital.

Mr. John Hunter, in the Haymarket.

Mr. J. O. Justamond, in Macclesfield Street, Soho.

Lectures on the Teeth.

Mr. W. Rae, at Mr. Hunter's lecture room in the Haymarket.

Natural Philosophy.

Mr. Walker, at his House in Great George Street, Hanover Square.

(See "Medical Register," 1783, by S. F. Simmons, p. 50.)

A LIST OF PERIODICAL PUBLICATIONS DEVOTED TO MEDICINE DURING THE REIGN OF GEORGE III

ANNALS OF MEDICINE. Edited by Andrew Duncan. Vols. 1–3. Edinburgh, 1796–1804.

ANNALS OF MEDICINE AND SURGERY. Vols. 1–2. London, 1817–18.

EDINBURGH MEDICAL AND SURGICAL JOURNAL. Established in 1805.

ESSAYS AND OBSERVATIONS. Vols. 1–3. Edinburgh, 1770–71.

LONDON MEDICAL JOURNAL. By a Society of Physicians. Vols. 1–11. London, 1781–90.

Dr. Simmons was the first editor.

LONDON MEDICAL REPOSITORY. Vols. 1–20. London, 1814–23. After 1823 it was continued as the LONDON MEDICAL AND SURGICAL JOURNAL, and survived until 1836. The title of Vol. 1 of the new series was the LONDON MEDICAL, SURGICAL, AND PHARMACEUTICAL JOURNAL, and in 1825 it became the LONDON MEDICAL REPOSITORY AND REVIEW.

LONDON MEDICAL, SURGICAL, AND PHARMACEUTICAL REPOSITORY. Vols. 1–29. London, 1814–28.

LONDON MEDICAL AND SURGICAL SPECTATOR. Vols. 1–2. London, 1808–9.

MEDICAL AND CHIRURGICAL REVIEW. Vols. 1–15. London, 1795–1807.

MEDICAL COMMENTARIES. Edited by Andrew Duncan. Edinburgh, 1780–95.

MEDICAL COMMUNICATIONS of the Society for Promoting Medical Knowledge. Vols. 1–2. London, 1784–90.

MEDICAL ESSAYS AND OBSERVATIONS. Vols. 1–5. 1737–44. Continued to 1757. Published in Edinburgh.

MEDICAL ESSAYS AND OBSERVATIONS. Abridged from Memoirs of the Royal Academy of Sciences, Paris. 4 vols. London, 1764.

MEDICAL FACTS AND OBSERVATIONS. A continuation of the LONDON MEDICAL JOURNAL. Vols. 1–8. London, 1791–1800.

MEDICAL MUSEUM. Vols. 1–3. London, 1763–4.

MEDICAL OBSERVATIONS AND ENQUIRIES. By a Society of Physicians of London. Vols. 1–6. London, 1757–1812.

MEDICAL AND PHILOSOPHICAL COMMENTARIES. By a Society of Physicians of Edinburgh. London, 1774–95.

MEDICAL AND PHYSICAL JOURNAL. London, 1799–1833. This Journal was re-named the LONDON MEDICAL AND PHYSICAL JOURNAL.

MEDICAL RECORD AND RESEARCHES. Selected from the Papers of a Private Medical Association. London, 1798.

MEDICAL SPECTATOR. Vols. 1–3. London, 1791–96.

NEW MEDICAL AND PHYSICAL JOURNAL. Or " Annals Medicine and Surgery and Collateral Branches." Vols. 1–10. London, 1810–15.

NEW LONDON MEDICAL JOURNAL. Vols. 1–2. London, 1792–93.

Society for the Improvement of Medical and Chirurgical Knowledge. Vols. 1–3. London, 1793–1812.

Transactions of the College of Physicians. Vols. 1–6. 1767–1820.

Transactions of the Medical Society.

Transactions of the Medico-Chirurgical Society.